Arthritis

Your Questions Answered

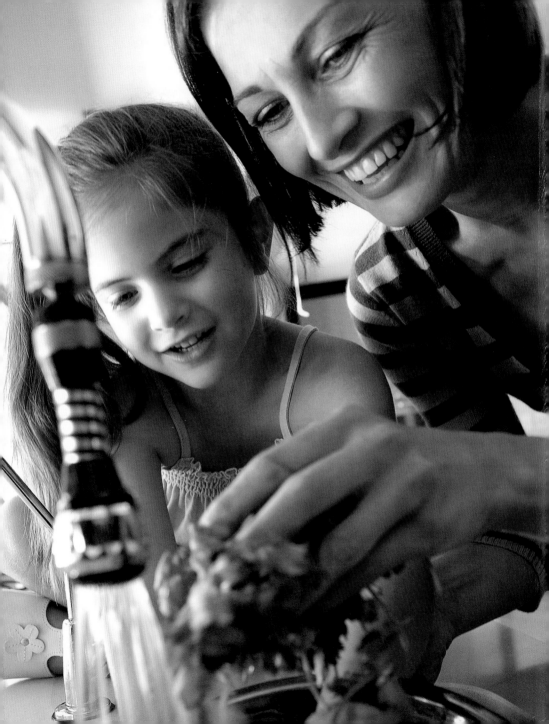

Arthritis

Your Questions Answered

Howard Bird, Caroline Green, Andrew Hamer,
Alison Hammond, Janet Harkness, Mike Hurley,
Paula Jefferson, Dorothy Pattison, David L. Scott

LONDON, NEW YORK, MUNICH, MELBOURNE, DELHI

DORLING KINDERSLEY
Editor Tom Broder
Senior Art Editor Nicola Rodway
US Senior Editor Jill Hamilton
Executive Managing Editor Adèle Hayward
Managing Art Editor Nick Harris
DTP Designer Traci Salter
Production Controller Freya Pugsley
Art Director Peter Luff
Publisher Corinne Roberts

DK INDIA
Senior Editor Dipali Singh
Project Editor Rohan Sinha
Editors Ankush Saikia, Aakriti Singhal
Project Designer Romi Chakraborty
DTP Coordinator Pankaj Sharma
DTP Designer Balwant Singh, Sunil Sharma
Head of Publishing Aparna Sharma

Edited for DK by Philip Morgan

First American Edition, 2007

Published in the United States by DK Publishing
375 Hudson Street, New York, New York 10014

07 08 09 10 11   10 9 8 7 6 5 4 3 2 1

AD325—April, 2007

Discover more at www.dk.com

Foreword

Arthritis is common—so common that many people think the problems associated with arthritis are a normal part of aging. Perhaps that is why they don't realize that things can be done to manage and control their arthritis. Although cures still elude us, many people lead normal lives despite their arthritis because of medical and surgical advances and lifestyle adjustments.

How do they do it? They take control. They participate in decisions that affect their arthritis care. They choose to learn about their disease—its physical effects on the body and the mental impact of a chronic condition. They learn about their options—exercise, diet, medical, surgical, even herbal—and the risks and benefits of each one. They also know what will improve if they choose to do nothing: Likely, nothing.

The choice is yours. Start with this book. Your healthcare provider will help you understand the answers and will work with you to find the best options given your personal health situation and your preferences. Live well despite your arthritis.

Robin K. Dore MD

Robin K. Dore MD
Clinical professor of medicine,
David Geffen School of Medicine at UCLA

Contents

The main types of arthritis

Understanding arthritis 10

Types of joint 14

Understanding osteoarthritis 16

Understanding rheumatoid arthritis 24

Understanding ankylosing spondylitis 32

Understanding gout 34

Pseudogout 37

Other types of arthritis?

Lupus 40

Polymyalgia rheumatica 42

Fibromyalgia 43

Localized soft-tissue disorders 47

Lower back pain 48

Carpal tunnel syndrome 53

Psoriatic arthritis 51

Infectious arthritis 54

Diagnosis and healthcare

Diagnosis 58

The healthcare team 63

Playing an active role in managing your arthritis 64

Complementary healthcare 70

Herbal medicines 72

Drug treatments

Taking medication 80

Analgesics and NSAIDs 83

Corticosteroids 87

Drug treatment of osteoarthritis 88

Drug treatment of rheumatoid arthritis 90

Common DMARDs 92

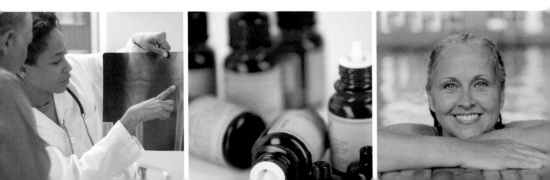

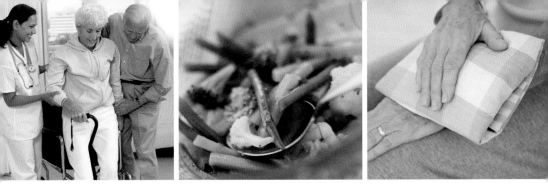

Surgical treatments
Surgical options **96**
Joint replacement **100**
Total knee and hip
    replacements **102**
Before and after surgery **104**
Returning home **109**

Living with arthritis
At work **116**
Asking for help **119**
At home **120**
Assistive devices **124**
Family life and caring for
    children **128**
Traveling and moving
    around **130**
Protecting your joints **132**
Coping with pain **136**
Coping with stress **140**
The ABCDE method **142**

Food and drink
Eating a healthy diet **146**
Nutrients to ease arthritis **151**
Helpful supplements **152**
Avoiding foods **157**
Weight control **160**

Physical activity
Getting enough exercise **164**
Maintaining mobility **171**
Neck exercises **172**
Leg and hip exercises **174**

Children with arthritis
Understanding juvenile
    arthritis **178**
Special needs **182**
Long-term outlook **183**

Useful addresses **184**
Index and acknowledgments **185**

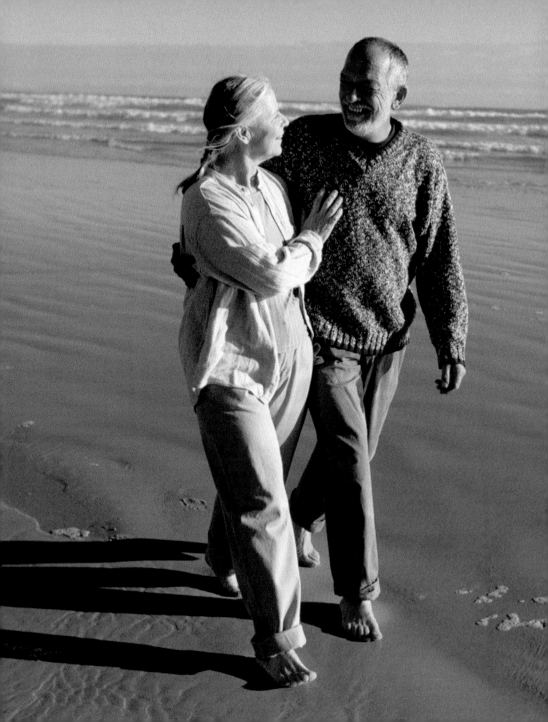

The main types of arthritis

Arthritis is very common, with more than 200 identifiable types that can be divided into 3 main groups: inflammatory arthritis, such as rheumatoid arthritis; noninflammatory arthritis, such as osteoarthritis; and regional or diffuse pain syndromes, such as fibromyalgia, which is a noninflammatory condition that causes pain in the muscles.

Understanding arthritis

Q What is arthritis?

Arthritis is a variety of many different conditions that can affect the joints at any stage of life, from the early days of childhood until the closing stages of old age. Arthritis develops for a number of reasons: wear and tear of the bones and cartilage in a joint; long-standing inflammation of the soft tissues around a joint; genetic predisposition; accumulation of crystals in a joint; and an infection in a joint. However, rheumatologists are uncertain about the causes of many types of arthritis.

Q What are the main challenges to overcome in arthritis?

People with arthritis often have to face difficulties that can compromise their way of life, although many can be overcome. There are a few main reasons for these challenges. First, the pain and inflammation may limit what you can do. Second, the progressive damage to your joints makes your muscles weak, making you less active. Third, the chronic pain wears you out and restricts the amount of exercise you are able to do. Finally, the conditions that are commonly associated with arthritis can put a strain on your quality of life.

Q What are the key characteristics of arthritis?

Arthritis has 2 key characteristics—joint pain and inflammation. Some people with arthritis have only pain but most have a combination of both. The hallmark of arthritis is joint inflammation, which leads to tenderness and swelling. People with arthritis usually complain of joint stiffness too. Symptoms vary enormously from person to person, depending on the type, extent, and severity of the arthritis.

Q Is the pain of arthritis the same in everybody?

No, the subjective sensation of pain in arthritis is very personal. It affects different people in different ways. People with arthritis usually seek medical advice because they want treatment to relieve the pain in their joints. The pain of arthritis can be chronic, which means that it is present most of the time and lasts for long periods. People with long-term pain experience all sorts of other effects, such as depression.

Q Does the nature of the pain help with diagnosing the type of arthritis?

No, not usually. Inflamed joints may be painful at rest and when they are moved. The pain of arthritis is normally associated with joint tenderness: when a joint is pressed it hurts. The more active the arthritis, the more joints are tender. The number of tender joints is one measure of the severity of the arthritis.

Q Why does arthritis make me so tired?

A marked feature of some types of arthritis is a sensation of unbearable fatigue. It is closely related to pain and to the reduction of mood, or even depression, that is common in arthritis. The fatigue is due to poor sleep, weakened muscles, and a disease process that may affect the whole body and mind.

Q How will arthritis affect the way I feel about myself?

A complex and subtle issue is the way arthritis can change your appearance and the way you look at yourself. How we look is of fundamental importance to us all. In the long term, arthritis affects both self-image and actual appearance, with consequent changes in self-perception. While these are difficult to quantify, they change a person's quality of life rather than cause a distinct disability, and are, therefore, important end results of arthritis.

Q **What is inflammation?**

When faced with an infection, irritation, or injury, the first response of your immune system is inflammation. Mast cells release histamine and other substances, increasing blood flow to the soft tissue in the joint and causing redness and heat. As blood vessels above the joint become wider, the blood vessels below it narrow, and the joint begins to swell. White blood cells accumulate in the affected area and release a variety of materials into the inflamed joint. The combination of the tissue swelling and the active substances from the white cells stimulates nerve endings and causes pain in the joint.

IDENTIFYING SYMPTOMS

Pain, inflammation, swelling, and stiffness are the key symptoms that doctors look for when trying to identify arthritis. Sometimes, these symptoms are accompanied by other features, such as loss of function and a sensation of unbearable fatigue, or general symptoms that affect the body as a whole.

SYMPTOMS	WHAT THEY MEAN
Pain	Pain in a joint or joints may be mild, moderate, or severe, and is usually chronic. Joint pain is a symptom of all types of arthritis.
Inflammation	Inflammation is a symptom of the various types of inflammatory arthritis, as well as many instances of osteoarthritis.
Swelling	Either the lining of the joint swells or fluid flows into the joint. Usually indicates inflammatory arthritis.
Stiffness	Morning stiffness that lasts for over an hour usually indicates a form of inflammatory arthritis. Stiffness that follows exercise or a period of inactivity usually suggests osteoarthritis.

Q **Which joints are affected?**

Most forms of arthritis affect the small joints in the hands and feet, and the large joints of the knees and hips, although any joint can be involved. When joints are painful, swollen, and stiff, they do not work well or move efficiently. Inflammation that persists can cause damage to an arthritic joint. Eventually, the damage becomes irreversible and the joints look distinctly different. Early stages of this condition differ in each type of arthritis and the specific joints affected, but the final common pathway of the damage leads to osteoarthritis (see p16) and joint failure.

Q **Is it just the joints that are affected?**

Damage to cartilage and bone is also accompanied by damage to tendons and soft tissues around joints. This may not be obvious at first, but later it can cause very typical abnormalities. Many forms of arthritis, particularly rheumatoid arthritis, are associated with changes in the skin or internal organs because they affect all the systems in the body, not just the joints. Sometimes, even the eyes are affected. However, osteoarthritis does not affect internal organs.

Q **Who is most likely to be affected by arthritis?**

Anyone can develop arthritis. It affects men and women of all ages, and sometimes children (see pp177–183). No one knows for sure why some people develop arthritis and not others, but there is a great deal of information about who is most at risk. Arthritis usually affects people in later life: about 60 percent of those over 85 years old are affected. This figure not only includes arthritis, especially osteoarthritis, which occurs mainly after middle age, but also arthritis developed at a younger age that has a cumulative and long-standing effect over time.

Types of joints

Joints are the sites in the body where two bones make contact. Some joints, such as the joints of the spine, are connected by disks of cartilage and permit some movement; others, such as the bones of the skull, are bound by fibrous tissue and permit no movement at all. Most joints have a space called the synovial cavity between the two bones. These synovial joints, such as the hip and elbow, allow movement and provide mechanical support. In general, the joints that allow movement are the joints affected by arthritis.

Although there are many types of synovial joint, they all share one underlying similarity: the surfaces of the two bones, where they meet, are covered in a thin superficial layer of tissue called the synovial membrane. Deeper layers of cartilage are able to absorb shocks. Synovial joints move in various ways. Some, such as the wrist, have a wide range of movement but do not move far in any direction. Hinge joints, such as the elbow, allow plenty of movement but only in a single plane. Ball-and-socket joints, such as the hip, have a wide range of movement in several directions.

A HEALTHY JOINT

The cartilage and synovial fluid play an important role in the health of a joint. The cartilage protecting the ends of the bones has to be smooth, springy, and tough. The fluid provides the nutrients the cartilage needs to renew itself and filters out the debris as the surface layers of cartilage are worn away. The movement of the joint constantly presses and releases the cartilage like a sponge, allowing nourishment to reach the deeper layers of cartilage and waste to be removed.

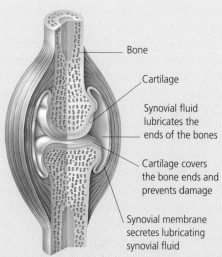

Bone

Cartilage

Synovial fluid lubricates the ends of the bones

Cartilage covers the bone ends and prevents damage

Synovial membrane secretes lubricating synovial fluid

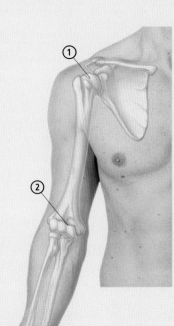

Movement in all directions

① **Ball-and-socket joint** The shoulder and hip are the two ball-and-socket joints in the body. One bone has a smooth, rounded end shaped like a ball, which fits into the cup-shaped socket of another bone. The joint allows movement in every direction.

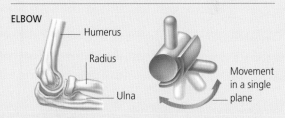

ELBOW
Humerus
Radius
Ulna
Movement in a single plane

② **Hinge joint** The knee, elbow, and finger joints are hinge joints. One bone has a cylindrical surface that fits into the groove of another bone. The joint allows a limb to bend and straighten.

Movement in several directions

③ **Saddle joint** The base of the thumb is the only saddle joint in the body. The metacarpal and trapezium bones have saddle-shaped ends that meet at right angles and allow movement in several directions with some rotation.

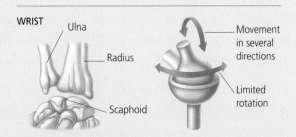

WRIST
Ulna
Radius
Scaphoid
Movement in several directions
Limited rotation

④ **Ellipsoidal joint** The wrist is an ellipsoidal joint in which the oval end of one bone fits into the cup of another. The joint allows movement in several directions but with only some rotation.

Understanding osteoarthritis

Q What is osteoarthritis?

Osteoarthritis is usually considered to be a degenerative condition involving wear and tear of the cartilage and bones where they meet at certain joints. There is more bony swelling and less soft-tissue swelling than in inflammatory arthritis and stiffness usually occurs at rest or after exercise.

Q How common is osteoarthritis?

Osteoarthritis is the most common form of arthritis. About 21 million people in the US have osteoarthritis, but only one-half of them actively seek treatment. The others never realize they have it, nor suffer any pain, although it shows up when people are X-rayed for other reasons. For most joints, especially those in the knees and the hands, osteoarthritis is more common—and also more severe—in women than in men.

Q What happens in osteoarthritis?

Osteoarthritis often develops slowly and varies from person to person. The surface of the cartilage in a joint breaks down and wears away, causing the bones to rub together. The results are pain, swelling, and reduced movement. Affected joints often stiffen after exercise. Eventually, the joint becomes deformed. Small spurs called osteophytes often form at the ends of the bones. Little pieces of cartilage or bone may break off and float inside the joint space, causing further pain and damage.

Q Which joints are most likely to be affected?

Osteoarthritis usually affects the top joints of the fingers and the base of the thumb, as well as the knees and the hips. However, any joint can be involved.

Q **Can osteoarthritis affect only one joint or does it always affect many joints?**

If you have osteoarthritis, you will probably find that only one joint, or a small number of joints, are affected. The most likely are the top joints of your fingers, the base joint of your thumb, your hips, or your knees.

JOINTS AFFECTED BY OSTEOARTHRITIS AND RHEUMATOID ARTHRITIS

Osteoarthritis and rheumatoid arthritis tend to affect certain joints, although any joint might be involved. The main joints affected by osteoarthritis are the hips, knees, hands, and feet. Osteoarthritis may affect the top and middle joints of the fingers and the base of the thumb. Rheumatoid arthritis targets a wider range of joints and varies considerably from one person to another. The hands (especially knuckles and the middle joints of the fingers) and feet are often involved, as are the wrists, ankles, shoulders, and knees. Less commonly affected are the elbows, jaws, and bones in the neck.

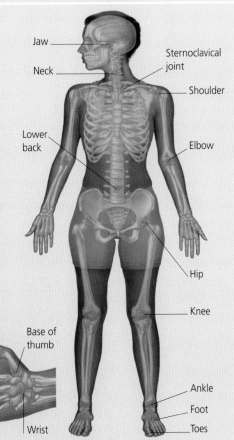

Jaw

Neck

Sternoclavical joint

Shoulder

Lower back

Elbow

Hip

Knee

Base of thumb

SKELETON

◻ Osteoarthritis

▨ Rheumatoid arthritis

Ankle

Foot

Wrist

Toes

Q Can I develop osteoarthritis at any age?

Age is the dominant risk factor of osteoarthritis, although younger people can also develop it following an injury. It usually starts after the age of 45 years and rises steeply with increasing age. Osteoarthritis is more common in the knee than in the hip. Taken together, the hips and knees are affected in 10–20 percent of people aged over 65 and are a major cause of pain and disability in elderly people. As more people live longer, osteoarthritis will become more common, because older people experience increasing muscle weakness and are less able to repair worn or damaged tissues.

Q Does inheritance play a role in osteoarthritis?

The presence of certain genes plays a role in the common form of nodal osteoarthritis (osteoarthritis affecting the finger joints), which particularly affects middle-aged women. In osteoarthritis of the knee and hip, heredity plays a smaller, yet significant role. General osteoarthritis probably has a genetic basis, too.

Q I have been diagnosed as obese—does this mean I am more at risk of developing osteoarthritis later in life?

Those people who weigh more than 25 percent above their target healthy weight are markedly more prone to osteoarthritis, particularly of the knee. At the same time, people who are overweight or obese increase their chances of osteoarthritis worsening once it has developed. Being overweight or obese can lead to osteoarthritis in several ways. First, being overweight increases the amount of force on weight-bearing joints, such as the knees. Second, the fatty tissues may alter the person's balance of hormones, which could affect cartilage and bone tissues. Third, obese people have relatively weak muscles, are less fit than people who are not overweight, and injure themselves more often.

Q I do a job that involves hard, physical work. Does this make me more predisposed to osteoarthritis?

Probably. If you repeatedly bend your knees (such as in squatting or heavy lifting), or have an occupation with an increased risk of injury to the knee joints, particularly a repetitive injury, then you are at risk of developing osteoarthritis of the knee later in life. Workers in industries such as forestry, construction, and agriculture are particularly at risk. Other joints may also be affected by overuse and repetitive injuries. See box, below, for advice on avoiding overuse injuries and excess wear.

AVOIDING INJURIES

If you regularly play sports or take part in an activity that requires repeated use of certain joints, you can reduce the risk of injuries or avoid them altogether by following a few key rules:

- Play the sport or practice the exercise that feels natural and enjoyable. If taking part in an activity makes you uncomfortable, you may increase the risk of getting injured.

- Buy the appropriate gear and equipment for your chosen sport or activity and you will feel much more comfortable. Don't struggle with worn-out or second-rate footwear, clothes, and equipment.

- Always warm up before you start, and cool down afterward.

- Try to build up the muscles around your joints.

- Try to exercise different muscles and joints and avoid activities that use one area of your body repetitively.

- Don't ignore the little stresses and strains in your body. If you feel pain, stop what you're doing.

- If you do sustain an injury, don't just ignore it and think it will be all right in the morning. Consult a doctor and get it examined so that it can heal properly.

Q **I play sports regularly—does this mean I am more likely to develop osteoarthritis in a joint later in life?**

Possibly. It depends on which joint is overused, the severity of the trauma, and the intensity of the inflammation that is produced as a result of the damage to cartilage and soft tissues. Repetitive trauma carries a high risk of future problems. One example is osteoarthritis of the knee that often develops in former professional soccer players, many of whom may have had knee replacement surgery at a relatively early age.

Q **Last winter I injured my knee while I was skiing—does this mean I may develop osteoarthritis later in life?**

Yes, it's possible, particularly if you damaged the cartilage. In addition, if you didn't wait for the injury to heal completely before you returned to physical exercise, you may have made it more likely for the joint to be affected by osteoarthritis—but it is difficult to say when this might occur.

Q **Is it true that a major injury to or surgery on a joint can lead to osteoarthritis?**

Yes. A major injury to, or surgery on, a joint may lead to osteoarthritis at that site later in life. Any hard and repetitive activity may injure a joint and make it prone to osteoarthritis. If you exercise too soon after a joint injury and before it has time to heal properly, the joint may also develop osteoarthritis.

Q **I'm a woman in my late 40s, expecting menopause at any time. Am I likely to develop osteoarthritis sooner or later?**

After menopause, a woman's body changes in many ways because her ovaries have stopped producing the hormones estrogen and progesterone. Among the many effects that this hormonal change appears to have is an increased risk of developing osteoarthritis, particularly of the knees and hands. As a result, osteoarthritis is much more common in women of this age (late 40s to early 50s) than men; a postmenopausal woman is also at an increased risk of developing osteoporosis.

Q Who is more likely to develop osteoarthritis of the knee?

People between their late 50s and early 70s, and usually women rather than men, are more likely to develop osteoarthritis of the knee. It generally affects both knees. You may have a higher chance of developing osteoarthritis of the knee if you are overweight, have osteoarthritis in another joint, or have had a previous injury or knee surgery, in particular cartilage removal. Often, however, there is no obvious cause. Pain is usually felt at the front and sides of the knee. In the later stages of osteoarthritis, the knees can become bent and deformed.

Q Who is more likely to develop osteoarthritis of the hip?

Women and men are equally affected by osteoarthritis of the hip in which mechanical wear and tear causes the cartilage of the joint to deteriorate. It can start in the 40s but it usually develops later in life. One or both hips are equally likely to be involved. Certain hip problems that were present at birth or have developed in childhood may later lead to osteoarthritis. Some people have anatomical features that predispose them to osteoarthritis. For example, in certain cases the acetabulum (the cup of the pelvic socket in which the head of the thighbone sits) is not as well developed as it should be.

Q Who is more likely to develop osteoarthritis of the hands?

Osteoarthritis of the hands mainly affects women and commonly starts in the late 40s or early 50s, often around the time of menopause. The condition chiefly affects the joint at the base of the thumb, and the joints at the top of the fingers. Although the fingers become knobbly and sometimes slightly bent, they usually continue to function well and rarely cause long-term problems.

Myth "Cold, wet weather makes osteoarthritis worse"

Truth Cold, wet weather may make your joints feel worse but there is no strong evidence to suggest that your osteoarthritis is affected. Particularly cold weather may affect the circulation of blood to the hands and feet, and this may make your joints feel stiff. People often think that moving to a warm, dry climate might improve their arthritis. However, osteoarthritis is just as common in warmer regions as in colder climates.

Q What is nodal osteoarthritis?

Nodal osteoarthritis affects the finger joints. These joints become swollen and tender, especially at the onset of the condition, and then develop firm, bony, knobby swellings. In some cases, similar bony swellings appear on the joints in the middle of the fingers.

Q How will osteoarthritis affect my mobility and flexibility?

This often depends on the time of day because pain and stiffness often appear in the morning and after exercise. It also depends on how advanced your condition is. Pain and stiffness will restrict the flexibility of your affected joints and your mobility will obviously be affected if you have osteoarthritis in your hip or knee.

Q What treatment will I need for osteoarthritis?

In the early stages, it is important to strengthen the muscles around an affected joint with exercise. Your doctor will probably prescribe analgesics and then recommend NSAIDs if analgesics fail to help or if there are inflammatory episodes accompanying your osteoarthritis. Supplements such as glucosamine and chondroitin (see p152), intra-articular injections, and topical counterirritants sometimes help (see p81). However, if your osteoarthritis is rapidly deteriorating in one joint, you may be advised to undergo surgery (usually successful) before damage at one joint puts strain on others and the problem becomes widespread.

Q What can I expect from my osteoarthritis in the long term?

Mild osteoarthritis (see p14) does not necessarily get worse and may remain relatively stable for the rest of your life. In later years, your mobility may be about the same as would be normal with the aging process. Symptoms tend to vary; you might find, for example, that stiffness and pain tend to be worse in the morning.

Understanding rheumatoid arthritis

Q What is rheumatoid arthritis?

Rheumatoid arthritis is a chronic disease that is characterized by persistent inflammation of a number of joints. Over a prolonged period of time, this inflammation results in irreversible joint damage. Although its cause is unknown, it is usually thought to be an autoimmune disease in which the body starts to attack itself—but the evidence for this is incomplete. More than 21 million people in the US have rheumatoid arthritis, making it the most common form of inflammatory arthritis.

Q What is most likely to trigger the start of rheumatoid arthritis?

Gender, genetics, and age are the most important risk factors. Others include heavy smoking, obesity, and a history of blood transfusions. In women, early menopause associated with low levels of reproductive hormones can be a factor.

Q What happens in rheumatoid arthritis?

The synovial membrane of one or more joints becomes inflamed, causing pain and swelling. Stiffness is usually present for 1–2 hours in the morning but in severe cases can persist all day. When inflammation spreads to the synovial sheaths that protect the tendons, there is progressive and usually irreversible damage to joints. Bony swellings appear and deformity develops as the damaged joints begin to fail. Muscles weaken due to lack of use and from the effects of generalized inflammation.

Q How does rheumatoid arthritis start?

Rheumatoid arthritis starts in different ways. Usually, it starts slowly, with intermittent pain and swelling in some joints, especially in the fingers, wrists, and feet. In perhaps 1 in 5 cases, the disease starts very suddenly: one day the individual is normal and the next many joints are painful, swollen, and stiff. In some people, the disease starts in less typical ways. For example, it may involve only a single joint. In others, the disease comes and goes repeatedly, often over several years, before becoming persistent. Occasionally, it starts with pain and stiffness around the shoulders, mimicking a condition called polymyalgia rheumatica (see p42).

Q How does rheumatoid arthritis progress?

The way the disease progresses is very variable. Some people have a mild disease with few problems and can live normal lives. For others, the disease may enter a period of sustained remission, without returning, or else follows an intermittent course, when flare-ups are followed by remissions that do not last long. Many people have chronic persistent arthritis, in which continuing disease activity is marked by added flare-ups from time to time. A few people develop a persisting, severe arthritis that remains active despite the best therapies.

Q Will I become disabled?

Inflammation and damage to joints together can cause marked disability. This varies with time and is unique to an individual, depending on how the joints are involved. Some people are simply unable to go back to their normal activities. The disability is also psychological and social. For example, many, though by no means all, people with rheumatoid arthritis find it difficult to work and some may need to leave their job as a result.

Q Can I develop rheumatoid arthritis at any age?

Rheumatoid arthritis can begin at any age. It was viewed traditionally as starting in young adulthood, with a peak age of onset between 20 and 45 years. For unknown reasons, this has changed and the average age of onset has increased to 60 years.

Q Are women more likely to be affected by rheumatoid arthritis than men?

Yes. About three-quarters of people with rheumatoid arthritis are women. Research studies suggest that in a population of 100,000 adults, there will be approximately 36 new cases of rheumatoid arthritis in women and 14 in men per year. However, the incidence of rheumatoid arthritis rises steeply as people grow older, especially in men.

Q As I approach menopause, am I likely to develop rheumatoid arthritis?

There is a greater risk that you will develop rheumatoid arthritis at menopause when your ovaries stop producing the hormones estrogen and progesterone. However, the relationship between these hormones and the development of autoimmune disorders such as rheumatoid arthritis is not well understood.

Q As a woman with rheumatoid arthritis, am I more likely to develop osteoporosis?

Women who have rheumatoid arthritis are more likely to develop osteoporosis. There may be several reasons for this link. First, the inflammation and pain may prevent or deter women from regular exercise, which can also have a negative effect on the strength of their bones. Second, studies show that rheumatoid arthritis can make you more susceptible to osteoporosis because of the bone loss that may occur around the affected joints. Finally, if you take corticosteroids (see p87) for the pain and inflammation, there is a significant risk of reduction in bone density.

Q If one of my parents developed rheumatoid arthritis, am I more likely to develop it, too?

Genes play a significant role in the development of rheumatoid arthritis. Up to 60 percent of the predisposition to rheumatoid arthritis is explained by genetic factors. The condition is strongly related to the presence of a protein on the surface of white blood cells (leucocytes) called HLA-DR4.

Q If a blood test reveals I have the HLA–DR4 gene, will I develop rheumatoid arthritis?

Not necessarily. Some people with the gene never develop rheumatoid arthritis. What scientists have discovered is that this gene is present in some people with rheumatoid arthritis but not others. Evidence suggests that people who have the HLA–DR4 gene have rheumatoid arthritis more severely and are more likely to have rheumatoid nodules and erosion of the bones within their joints. Since the gene is important in determining how the immune system works, scientists thought they were on the verge of a breakthrough. To date, they have been unable to unravel the story further. As a result, the knowledge that someone has the HLA-DR4 gene has not yet influenced treatment.

Q Which joints are more likely to be affected by rheumatoid arthritis?

Rheumatoid arthritis targets a wider range of joints than osteoarthritis and varies considerably from one person to another. It often affects the same joints similarly, but not always simultaneously, on both sides of the body. Several specific joints are more commonly involved than others (see p17). In the hand, these include the base of the thumb, the middle joints of the fingers, the knuckles, and the wrists. The feet are often involved too, as are the ankles, shoulders, and knees. Less commonly affected are the elbows, jaws, and bones in the neck.

Myth "Rheumatoid arthritis affects only the joints"

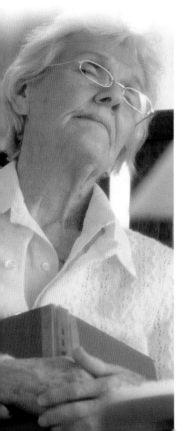

Truth Inflammatory arthritis affects other parts of the body, too. Rheumatoid nodules may appear on the skin due to prolonged pressure at various sites, such as elbows. The eyes and mouth may become dry while inflammation of the blood vessels may cause damage to the organs served by them, such as the heart and lungs. People with rheumatoid arthritis experience a general feeling of being unwell, an overwhelming fatigue, and depression.

Q What treatment will I need for rheumatoid arthritis?

In the very early days of your condition, NSAIDs (see p84) may provide you with some relief from your symptoms. However, while NSAIDs mask the symptoms, they do not prevent progressive joint damage. Such damage is best prevented by disease-modifying antirheumatoid drugs (see pp90–93). If you don't respond to these, you may be considered for a new generation of drugs called biologic agents (see p93), which specifically block the chemical messenger that causes rheumatoid arthritis in the early stages.

Q Will I have to go into the hospital for treatment?

Both the disease-modifying antirheumatoid drugs (DMARDs) and the biologic agents are extremely potent, so your treatment will be based in a hospital. Many hospitals also have "early arthritis" clinics: there is some evidence to indicate that if your rheumatoid arthritis is treated aggressively within the first 6 months, it is less severe, although it would perhaps be overly optimistic to suggest that it could be cured. As a last resort, you could be a candidate for surgery—either to remove the lining of a joint, resurface a joint, or replace a joint.

Q How will rheumatoid arthritis affect my mobility and flexibility?

The symptoms of rheumatoid arthritis mysteriously appear and disappear. When they reappear, the symptoms of inflammation, swelling, pain, and stiffness flare up, reducing the flexibility of the affected joints and restricting your ability to move. The elderly have weaker muscles than younger people, so they find it tougher to cope. It is harder for them to maintain strength and fitness through exercise, so their disability is likely to increase. Their movement can be further restricted by joint or bone damage due to a fracture caused by a fall.

Q **What can I expect from rheumatoid arthritis in the long term?**

Most people with rheumatoid arthritis have variable symptoms. The arthritis is active for weeks and months, then dies down or disappears for a while before flaring up again. The amount of damage to the joints depends on the severity of flare-ups and how often they occur. Eventually, you are likely to have some degree of permanent damage. However, the chances are that you will live relatively normally, and it is important to realize that severe disability is uncommon. Very rarely, flare-ups cease altogether; but if this happens, any joint damage will remain.

Q **If the treatment for rheumatoid arthritis is effective, will it continue to remain the same or will I have to make changes?**

You may be taking a drug that suits you and has kept your symptoms well controlled for many years. But sometimes, for reasons that are not related to your arthritis, this drug may stop being an option. From midlife onward, other health problems start to become more common. In some cases, your arthritis drugs may make them worse or they may require medication that interacts with your existing treatment. For example, if you develop hypertension (high blood pressure), you may not be able to take steroids to reduce inflammation, because they raise blood pressure. If you develop a kidney or liver disease, you will not be able to take some DMARDs because their potential side effects include damage to the kidneys or liver. If you do need to discontinue an arthritis drug or to take a mixture of drugs for different conditions, your doctor will tell you what is best for your situation. In some cases, you may need to take drugs for a possibly life-threatening disease at the expense of controlling your arthritis. It is all a question of balance.

Q How do elderly people with rheumatoid arthritis cope with the toxicity of drugs?

Drugs for treating arthritis tend to have a more toxic effect in elderly people. This is partly because the older we get, the less efficient our bodies become at breaking down drugs. Also, older people are more likely to be taking drugs for other conditions and these may interact with arthritis drugs. For this reason, doctors keep the dosages to a minimum and carefully monitor their older patients to watch for reactions.

Q Does rheumatoid arthritis put me at greater risk of developing other diseases in the long term?

Possibly. Research studies suggest that conditions such as heart disease, osteoporosis, stroke, and infections may be more likely. One reason may be that people with rheumatoid arthritis are not able to exercise freely. In some cases, the drugs for rheumatoid arthritis can raise blood pressure (a risk factor for stroke) or weaken the immune system, making infections more likely.

REDUCING THE RISK OF LONG-TERM PROBLEMS

There are a number of ways of looking after yourself so that you minimize and reduce the risks of developing long-term problems of rheumatoid arthritis.

- Take an active part in managing your arthritis.
- Stay physically active. Maintain your mobility and exercise your joints and muscles regularly (see p164).
- Eat a well-balanced diet (see p146).
- Keep your weight to a healthy level (see p160).
- Don't smoke or drink excessively.
- Follow your doctor's instructions and take medication.
- Make sure you are tested and monitored regularly so that problems can be treated early.

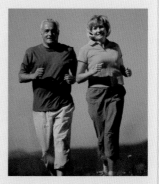

Understanding ankylosing spondylitis

Q **What is ankylosing spondylitis?**

This inflammatory disease predominantly affects the spine and can result in marked stiffness or even fusion of the spine. "Ankylosing" is another word for stiffening, while "spondylitis" means inflammation of the spine. The cause of ankylosing spondylitis is unknown. However, a gene called HLA-B27 plays a role in the condition and up to 95 of 100 people with this condition have this gene. Some studies estimate 1 in 1,000 adults have ankylosing spondylitis, while others suggest that a mild version of the disease affects up to 1 in 100 adults.

Q **Are men more likely to develop ankylosing spondylitis?**

Yes, particularly men in their 20s and 30s. The ratio of men to women with ankylosing spondylitis is about 5 to 1. When the disease affects women, it tends to be milder.

Q **Which joints are more likely to be affected by ankylosing spondylitis?**

The joints between the vertebrae of the spine become inflamed, starting at the sacroiliac joints, the two joints that connect the sacrum at the base of the spine with the pelvis. The ligaments around the joints accumulate calcium salts and become hard. New bone forms once the inflammation subsides and, as a result, the vertebrae become deformed and the spine stiffens and becomes inflexible. Eventually, in severe cases, the joints may fuse and prevent movement. The joints connecting the vertebrae to the ribs may become inflamed, making breathing difficult.

Q **What happens in ankylosing spondylitis?**

The initial features are stiffness, an ache in the lower back, and reduced movement of the spine. Stiffness is present in the morning and often lasts for several hours. Some people have only mild aches and pains that progress slowly over months or years. Others have a more active disease that leads to potential weight loss and feelings of ill-health and fatigue. The disorder is also associated with iritis (inflammation of the iris), with symptoms such as an acutely inflamed red eye, which requires immediate medical attention to avoid permanent eye damage.

Q **How will ankylosing spondylitis affect my mobility and flexibility?**

Over time, the disease may clear up or cause only minor stiffness; or it may become more serious as the stiffness progresses, with limited movement of the spine resulting in a hunched posture, rounded spine, and a flat chest. Arthritis of other joints, such as the hip, usually clears up with time. Only a few patients develop a progressive destructive arthritis of their joints.

Q **What treatment will I need for ankylosing spondylitis?**

Regular exercise or physical therapy are good for combating stiffness, while the best drugs are DMARDs (see pp90–93) such as methotrexate, sulfasalazine, and possibly leflunomide. There is increasing evidence that biologic agents (see p93) that block the chemical involved in triggering ankylosing spondylitis are also effective. Injectable gold and cyclosporine are only partially effective.

Q **What is the long-term outlook?**

The outlook for most people with ankylosing spondylitis is good. Severe disability is unusual because treatment (especially regular exercise or physical therapy) is very effective in preventing joint stiffness. You have a reasonable chance of being only mildly affected in your daily life.

Understanding gout

Q What is gout?

Gout is an inflammatory arthritis with a clearly identified cause—the presence of uric acid crystals in the synovial fluid of a joint. Gout is a disorder of the body's uric acid metabolism and affects the joints, particularly the big toe, where it can be very painful. In fact, during an acute attack, this condition can be the most painful arthritis of all. It is generally related to various lifestyle factors, such as eating processed meats and drinking excessive amounts of alcohol.

Q How common is gout?

Gout affects approximately 2.1 million adults in the US and usually develops in middle age. The frequency of gout increases with age. The condition is about 3 times more common in men than in women; gout rarely affects women before they reach menopause.

Q What is most likely to trigger the start of gout?

Gout can be triggered by illness, surgery, trauma, or a metabolic disturbance. Dramatic weight gain or loss or sudden changes in diet can sometimes trigger an attack. Gout often seems to come on for no obvious reason, but an attack is usually preceded by a period of high uric acid levels in the blood.

Q What happens in an attack of gout?

Acute gout causes agony. There is a sudden onset of pain in a single joint, which is hot, red, and very tender to the touch. The initial attack will usually resolve within around 10 days, but may recur. Some people have intermittent recurrent episodes; in others, gout is like rheumatoid arthritis, becoming chronic and destructive.

Q **My father developed gout—does this mean I am more likely to develop it?**

Not necessarily. Gout does sometimes run in the family, but if you are a male and drink excessive amounts of alcohol, your chances of inheriting the condition will be higher than if you are a female and a teetotaller. Evidence shows that many people with gout have an inherited tendency for their uric acid levels to be high.

Q **Can cancer treatment and antihypertensive drugs make gout more likely?**

Uric acid levels may increase after medical treatment. Cancer treatment causes cells to be broken down and purines (nitrogen-containing compounds) released from DNA. Thiazide diuretics, such as hydrochlorothiazide for hypertension, also raise uric acid levels.

Q **Does everyone with high uric acid levels in their blood develop gout?**

No. And curiously, many patients who experience an acute attack of gout do not have raised uric acid levels. Nevertheless, it is true to say that the higher the uric acid levels, the more likely the chance of an attack of gout.

Q **How do the levels of uric acid become so high?**

Most of the uric acid comes from within the body as a natural waste product, created when purines and proteins are broken down. Uric acid is normally excreted in urine, but when the balance between the amount produced and the amount excreted is upset, levels of uric acid in the blood start to rise. When the levels become too high, crystals form and collect in the white cells in joints and other tissues. This can cause acute arthritis with intense local pain.

Q **Which of my joints are more likely to be affected by gout?**

Gout most commonly and traditionally targets the joint at the base of the big toe where the pain is also the most excruciating. Others joints that can be affected include the elbows, knees, ankles, wrists, and hands.

Q Why are attacks of gout so painful?

In gout, high levels of uric acid in the blood cause crystals of uric acid to accumulate in the synovial fluid and joint capsule of one or more joints. These crystals are sharp, like needles. In an attack of gout, which may come without warning, the pain can be unbearable. The affected joint turns red with inflammation and swells up.

Q Will the crystals that cause gout affect other parts of my body?

The sharp, needlelike crystals also accumulate in other parts of the body—for example, under the skin where the white deposits are known as tophi. These tophi are conventionally on the earlobes and elbows, but they can occur at many sites, including the soft tissues of the hands and feet. Crystals may also accumulate in the kidneys, where they form stones and can cause renal failure.

Q Should I stop eating red meat and drinking alcohol?

Perhaps it would be a good idea, especially if your uric acid levels are sometimes shown to be high. Some of the uric acid that contributes to gout comes from a high intake of purines, which are essential nitrogen compounds found in lentils, dried beans, sardines, shellfish, and organ meats. So removing these from your diet may help keep your uric acid levels low.

Q What treatment will I need for gout?

Analgesics and anti-inflammatory agents have a role in managing acute attacks of gout. Long-term treatment is with drugs that alter uric acid metabolism. The most commonly used drug for this purpose is allopurinol. Other drugs include colchicine and corticosteroids (see p87).

Pseudogout

Q What is pseudogout?

Like gout, acute arthritis can be caused when crystals of calcium pyrophosphate dihydrate are deposited in joints, particularly the knee and less often the big toe. This is known as pseudogout because of its similarity to gout. Pseudogout affects more men than women when compared with gout, but it usually occurs later in life. It may also run in families. In some people, the symptoms of pseudogout are very similar to those in rheumatoid arthritis and osteoarthritis. The crystals may collect in the cartilage around joints, especially in elderly people, without causing symptoms. Many elderly people with osteoarthritis can develop pseudogout when the crystals interact with their condition.

Q Where do the crystals of calcium pyrophosphate dihydrate come from?

The exact source of the crystals and why they cause acute arthritis are unknown. There may be a link with abnormal connective tissue or cartilage, or with other disorders, such as an underactive thyroid gland, excess iron storage, an overactive parathyroid gland, and other causes of excess calcium in the blood. Episodes of pseudogout can follow surgery, metabolic disturbances, or an injury to a joint.

Q How is pseudogout treated?

You can take analgesics and NSAIDs to relieve the pain, reduce swelling, and ease the stiffness. But they do not prevent further damage to the affected joint. Your doctor may recommend the removal of fluid from the joint and may inject corticosteroids to alleviate the inflammation. You should also exercise the joint regularly to strengthen the surrounding muscles.

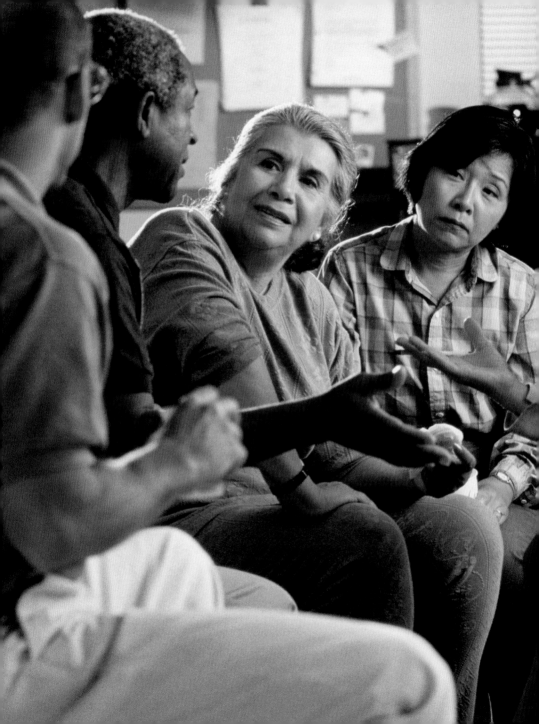

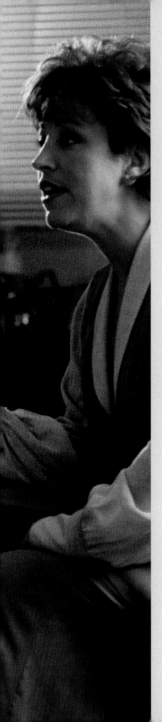

Other types of arthritis

Many conditions involving joint pain or inflammation of soft tissues and other areas of the body may be related to arthritis. Other disorders, such as vasculitis and carpal tunnel syndrome, may accompany different types of arthritis. If you have arthritis, you may be at a slightly increased risk of developing such disorders, but they are not an inevitable progression; any of them can also affect people who do not suffer from arthritis.

Lupus

Q What is lupus?

Systemic lupus erythematosus (SLE), or lupus for short, is a disorder of the immune system that causes inflammation in the connective tissues in many parts of the body. Lupus is highly variable. Many people are affected mildly while others may have severe symptoms that intermittently flare up and then subside for long periods. Permanent improvement is very rare.

Q What are the symptoms of lupus?

The first symptoms are often aches and pain in the joints, particularly in the hands and feet. Another major symptom is a red skin rash, which typically spreads across the nose and cheeks—this is called the butterfly rash. In addition, depression and a feeling of general fatigue are common.

Q How common is lupus?

Lupus is a relatively uncommon disorder. Its frequency varies depending on age, gender, and ethnicity—which reflects the impact of genetic risk factors. Overall, it is seen in about 1 or 2 adults in 1,000. It is most common in African–American women, about 21 in 1,000. There are about 40 new cases per million each year. Lupus can take several years to be diagnosed after symptoms first appear.

Q Who is most at risk of lupus?

The disease is far more common in women than in men, and is also more likely to occur in women of African–American and Asian origin. Women with lupus should consult their doctor if they are thinking of conceiving. Lupus is comparatively rare in children and does not usually develop in adults once they have reached the age of 50 unless it is due to a medication.

Q What is most likely to trigger the start of lupus?

It is not known what triggers the disease but viral infections, stress, and hormone imbalances may be involved. Certain drugs can occasionally cause side effects that resemble the symptoms of lupus.

Q I have a very red skin rash on my leg—could it be a symptom of lupus?

It could be. A blotchy red rash on the skin is a common feature of lupus and can appear anywhere on the body. The skin rashes tend to become worse if they are exposed to sunlight or ultraviolet radiation. In some instances, sunlight may even act as a trigger and cause the disease to flare up.

Q Does lupus affect other parts of the body apart from the joints?

The areas affected by lupus may include the skin and the tissues of the lungs, heart, and kidneys. The nervous system is sometimes involved, too. Some people develop persistent mouth ulcers and experience hair loss. Inflammation of the lining of the heart and lungs can cause chest pain and shortness of breath. If the kidneys are affected, serious complications may arise, such as high blood pressure and kidney failure, but these are rare.

Q How is lupus treated?

A number of different drugs can be used, all of which suppress the immune system and are, therefore, often termed immunosuppressive drugs. Azathioprine is commonly used, while hydroxychloroquine is helpful for mild cases. Other treatments include cyclosporin and mycophenolate mofetil. If severe vasculitis (inflammation of the blood vessels) is present, the condition may need to be treated with systemic corticosteroid therapy, with or without the potent anticancer drug cyclophosphamide. This therapy is conducted under strict medical supervision because of the side effects involved.

Polymyalgia rheumatica

Q What is polymyalgia rheumatica?

In this disorder, pain and stiffness affect many muscles, mainly in the neck and shoulders, and around the hips, and thighs. The symptoms can develop gradually or rapidly, and may include fever, night sweats, depression, and general fatigue and weakness. Polymyalgia rheumatica affects only about 5 adults in 1,000. It is rare under the age of 50 years; its frequency increases with age and it is most common in elderly women.

Q What is most likely to trigger the start of polymyalgia rheumatica?

Polymyalgia rheumatica is triggered by an abnormal immune response; this may follow a viral infection. It may also follow other infections such as pneumonia caused by the microorganism mycoplasma. Genetic risks are important, and these are similar to those influencing rheumatoid arthritis (see pp24–31).

Q Are there any other problems associated with polymyalgia rheumatica?

In some people, it is associated with giant cell arteritis, a form of blood vessel inflammation caused by an immune response. This affects arteries in the head—most often the temporal arteries beneath the skin of the temples, and those in the neck in the elderly—causing headaches.

Q How is polymyalgia rheumatica treated?

Polymyalgia rheumatica is usually treated with drugs to relieve pain and reduce inflammation. If giant cell arteritis is involved, it needs rapid treatment because serious complications can cause permanent blindness in one or both eyes. Drugs to reduce inflammation are usually effective, although some people need to take corticosteroids for several years to control it.

Fibromyalgia

Q What is fibromyalgia?

The term fibromyalgia describes a collection of symptoms, the most important of which is persistent pain in many areas of the body. Fibromyalgia affects the muscles and other connective tissues, such as tendons and ligaments, and is not a joint disorder as such.

Q How common is fibromyalgia?

Fibromyalgia is a common problem that affects about 1 or 2 in 100 adults, mostly women. Milder symptoms, often termed chronic widespread pain, affect up to 4 in 100 adults. Many people with fibromyalgia also have associated medical disorders such as irritable bowel syndrome and headache.

Q Who is most at risk of fibromyalgia?

About 9 in every 10 people with fibromyalgia are women over the age of 40. Although the cause of fibromyalgia is not known, it may be linked to stress, anxiety, or depression.

Q What happens in fibromyalgia?

The pain of fibromyalgia may occur anywhere, often on both sides of the body at once, and is usually experienced as widespread aching and stiffness. Typically, several small sites in particular areas, such as at the base of the skull and around the shoulder blades and breastbone, are painful when pressed. Doctors use the number and distribution of these "tender points" to diagnose fibromyalgia (see box, p44). Although this disorder may persist for many months or years, it does not cause damage to muscles or joints and will not lead to the development of arthritis or make existing arthritis worse.

TENDER POINTS

Fibromyalgia can be difficult to diagnose, so doctors rely on the presence of tender points, located in 9 symmetrical pairs, at particular sites around the body. Although this technique is not foolproof because tenderness can vary from day to day, fibromyalgia may be confirmed if 11 of the 18 points are tender when pressed. The pairs of tender points can be found at the following locations: at the base of the skull, at the base of the neck, on top of the shoulders, on the inside edge of the shoulder blades, below the elbows, at the top of the breastbone, at low back, at the top of the outer thighs, and on the fat pad just above the inside of the knees.

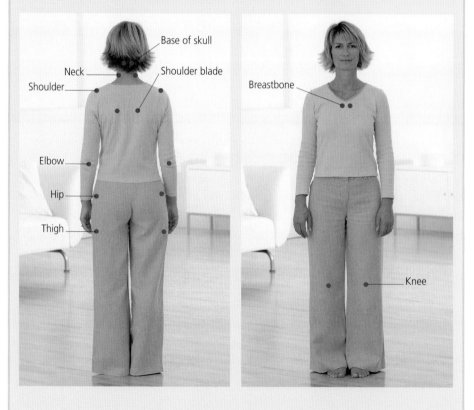

Base of skull
Neck
Shoulder blade
Shoulder
Breastbone
Elbow
Hip
Thigh
Knee

Q Does fibromyalgia affect other parts of the body?

About 9 in 10 people with fibromyalgia are affected by severe fatigue and have problems sleeping. Other associated symptoms include headaches, irregular bowel movements that alternate between diarrhea and constipation (known as irritable bowel syndrome), and a frequent need to urinate.

Q How is fibromyalgia treated?

Fibromyalgia can be difficult to treat, although the symptoms may be eased in various ways. For example, analgesics may bring some relief and your doctor may prescribe low-dose antidepressants to improve disturbed sleep. Antidepressants taken at night, in a dose much lower than that normally needed to relieve depression, significantly modify the symptoms of fibromyalgia during the day. The tricyclic antidepressant drug amitriptyline has been succeeded by trazadone, and a variety of SSRIs (selective serotonin reuptake inhibitors) also display promise in treating this condition. Self-help measures, such as low-impact exercise (see below) and applying gentle heat to painful areas (see p138), may also help.

Q How can exercise help relieve the pain of fibromyalgia?

Gentle exercise, such as walking, swimming, or cycling, for 15–20 minutes a day can help people with fibromyalgia. There is also good evidence to suggest that aerobic exercise (moderate to high intensity) can help, too. Regular exercise improves the condition of the heart, circulation, and muscles of the body; it also reduces pain and other symptoms. Exercise also stimulates the body to produce growth hormone (secreted by the pituitary gland), which can be low in people with fibromyalgia.

Myth "You only get tennis elbow by playing tennis"

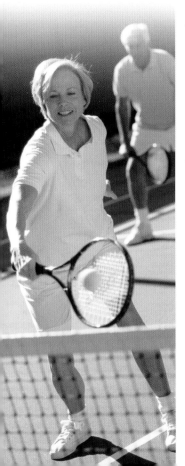

Truth   This condition, in which the outer part of the elbow is inflamed and painful, is not necessarily due to playing tennis. Known medically as lateral epicondylitis, it often occurs when strenuous repetitive movements, such as those used in heavy manual work, cause tiny tears in the tendon. The condition may also be caused by a direct blow to the arm, or may be a complication of arthritis.

Localized soft-tissue disorders

Q My elbow is really tender and painful— is this what they call tennis elbow?

It could be, especially if the pain and tenderness is around the bony point of the elbow and involves stiffness. The pain is caused by damage to the tendon connecting the muscles of the forearm to the upper arm bone (humerus). Continuous overuse of the arm may cause further damage.

Q What should I do to treat my tennis elbow?

For mild tennis elbow, rest the arm, apply ice packs to the painful area, and take anti-inflammatory drugs. For more severe damage, your doctor may suggest physical therapy. If the condition does not improve within a few weeks, your doctor may inject a corticosteroid into the tissue around your elbow joint.

Q There's a severe stabbing pain in the heel of my left foot when I first stand up in the morning—is this plantar fasciitis?

It might be, especially if you have injured the band of tough fibrous tissue called the plantar fascia on your sole. Plantar fasciitis occurs when an area of this tissue becomes inflamed where it attaches to the calcaneus bone of the heel. Older people are prone to this because the tissues in their feet lose some elasticity and their heels absorb less shock. Sitting down brings only temporary relief. The main risk factors are sudden weight gain and existing foot problems, such as flat feet and high arches.

Q How can my plantar fasciitis be treated?

Your doctor may suggest drugs to reduce inflammation. However, doing gentle stretching exercises and wearing an arch support in your shoe may also help.

Lower back pain

One of the most common health complaints in adults, lower back pain can have many causes, but is usually the result of a minor injury to the soft tissues of the back. An acute pain in the lower back that develops suddenly is often due to a physical activity, such as lifting a heavy weight, that puts excess strain on muscles or tendons. Such an injury can cause a sharp pain in one place or a more widespread, dull ache, as well as stiffness when you bend down.

Another cause of back pain is a condition commonly known as a "slipped disk," in which one of the shock-absorbing pads of cartilage between two vertebrae is displaced (prolapsed) or damaged. If the disk presses against one of the spinal nerves, you may experience severe pain, as well as numbness and tingling in one leg. Persistent lower back pain and sciatica are frequently related to some types of arthritis, such as osteoarthritis or ankylosing spondylitis, that affect the joints of the spine.

SLIPPED DISK

Disks of cartilage separate the vertebrae in the spine. Each disk has a tough outer layer and a gel-like center. When a disk protrudes, it moves (slips) and presses against the spinal cord or on a spinal nerve, causing pain.

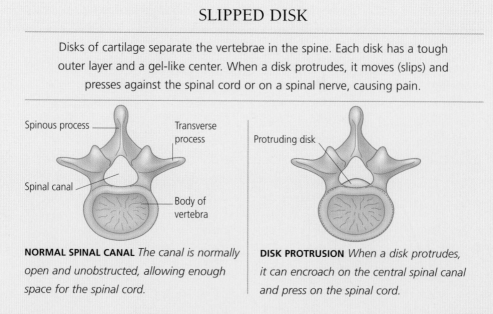

Spinous process

Transverse process

Protruding disk

Spinal canal

Body of vertebra

NORMAL SPINAL CANAL *The canal is normally open and unobstructed, allowing enough space for the spinal cord.*

DISK PROTRUSION *When a disk protrudes, it can encroach on the central spinal canal and press on the spinal cord.*

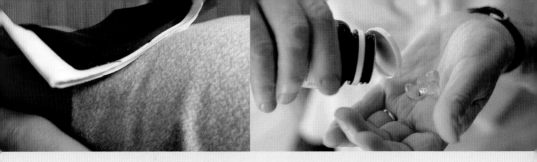

TREATING LOWER BACK PAIN

Back pain due to minor tissue damage usually clears up within a couple of weeks. Your doctor may suggest that you take analgesics, and you could try self-help measures, such as applying a heat pad or an ice pack to your back, to ease the symptoms. Bed rest may help if you are in severe pain, but do not prolong it for more than a day or two. If you suddenly have an acute attack of lower back pain, stay calm and don't panic. Just relax and breathe deeply. Keep your spine straight to take the weight off the disks of cartilage. Lie down or sit, whichever is the most comfortable, and rest. Contact your doctor if the pain does not ease up.

INCIDENCE OF BACK PAIN

Statistics show that back problems, such as lower back pain, are most likely to cause you trouble between the ages of 30 and 50 years, when the disks between your vertebrae contain more of the gel than in elderly people.

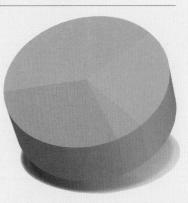

Approximately 25 percent of the population go through life without experiencing back pain.

About 40 percent have had back pain but are not suffering now.

About 30 percent of the population have back pain but do not seek medical help.

Only 5 percent of those who experience back pain receive treatment.

Q My knee is stiff and painful to move—is this bursitis?

It could well be, especially if you have put your knee through persistent and repeated movements or pressure. Inflammatory arthritis can also make you more susceptible to bursitis. When the fluid-filled sac, or bursa, that cushions your knee becomes inflamed and tender, the joint turns stiff and painful to move. Less often, bursitis may be caused by an infection as well. It commonly affects the elbow and shoulder.

Q What can I do to relieve my bursitis?

Resting the joint, applying ice-packs, and taking anti-inflammatory drugs often relieve the symptoms, which usually last a week. If the bursitis recurs or remains troublesome, your doctor may suggest draining the bursa.

Q I feel as if a tendon in my shoulder is particularly painful—is this tendinitis?

It could be, especially if you have injured or strained the tendon. In tendinitis, the synovium (a sheath of tissue surrounding the tendon) often becomes inflamed at the same time; this accompanying disorder is known as tenosynovitis. Tendinitis and tenosynovitis cause pain and stiffness around a joint; the area may be swollen, red, and warm to touch. Tendons in the shoulder, elbow, knee, and heel are most likely to be affected.

Q How can I treat the tendinitis in my shoulder?

The treatment of tendinitis includes appropriate rest to allow the inflammation to settle as well as local measures, such as the use of heat and cold (see p138), analgesics, and anti-inflammatory drugs, to reduce inflammation. You may need physical therapy, too. Over-the-counter analgesics, such as acetaminophen, and nonsteroidal anti-inflammatory drugs (NSAIDs), such as ibuprofen, may help; ask your doctor if it is okay to take these. Also avoid straining your shoulder.

Carpal tunnel syndrome

Q **My left wrist hurts and the hand feels numb and has a tingling sensation. What's wrong?**

You may have developed carpal tunnel syndrome. In this condition, the main nerve from the forearm to the hand is compressed as it passes through the wrist, causing numbness and tingling in the hand (see box, p52). You may feel pain in your wrist and up your forearm, too.

Q **What happens in carpal tunnel syndrome?**

The cause of carpal tunnel syndrome is not always obvious, but it is sometimes linked to repetitive hand movements that cause swelling of the soft tissues within the carpal tunnel. This is why carpal tunnel syndrome is sometimes a form of repetitive strain injury. Damage to the joints of the wrist, due to injury or arthritis, may also cause narrowing of the carpal tunnel. Many people find that their symptoms are most severe during the night or when they wake in the morning. Without treatment, carpal tunnel syndrome may eventually lead to permanent numbness in the hand, wasting of muscles, and a weakened grip.

Q **How can my carpal tunnel syndrome be treated?**

Wearing a wrist splint brings relief (see p123). Some people claim that practicing a yoga pose called namaste, in which the palms are held together in front of the chest, with the elbows pointing out to the sides, may also help (see box, p52). If the symptoms are particularly bad, your doctor may prescribe anti-inflammatory drugs. In some cases, surgery to cut the carpal ligament and enlarge the carpal tunnel may help relieve pressure on the median nerve.

PAIN IN THE WRIST

The carpal tunnel is the gap between the wrist bones (carpals). The median nerve passes through the tunnel, underneath a band of ligament, and branches into nerves that serve the fingers and the thumb. These nerves control some of the muscles of the hand. In carpal tunnel syndrome, pressure on the median nerve causes numbness and a tingling sensation, particularly in the first and middle fingers and the thumb.

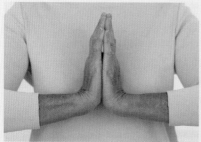

NAMASTE POSE A yoga pose called namaste can bring relief to the pain of carpal tunnel syndrome. The palms are held together in front of the chest, with the elbows pointing out to the sides.

THE CARPAL TUNNEL

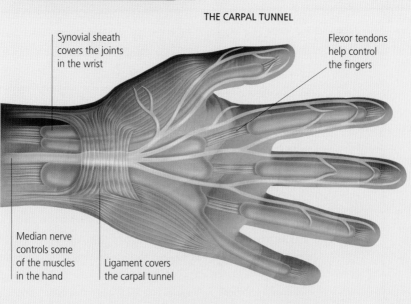

Synovial sheath covers the joints in the wrist

Flexor tendons help control the fingers

Median nerve controls some of the muscles in the hand

Ligament covers the carpal tunnel

Psoriatic arthritis

Q What is psoriatic arthritis?

Psoriatic arthritis is an inflammatory arthritis frequently associated with the skin condition psoriasis. Sometimes, however, the arthritis develops first. The condition is not common. About 1 in 50 people has psoriasis; of these, about 1 in 14 develops psoriatic arthritis. It affects both men and women, and usually starts in middle age. Psoriatic arthritis is an autoimmune disorder, which means that it occurs because the body's own immune system attacks the joints. The exact cause is unknown, although genetics play a small part. Like ankylosing spondylitis, it may be triggered by a bacterial infection.

Q Which joints are more likely to be affected by psoriatic arthritis?

The neck, shoulders, elbows, wrists, knees, ankles, base of the spine, and all the joints of the hands and feet are likely to be affected. Many people experience inflammation in one or two joints. In others, it involves the top joint of the fingers or toes, with pitting, discoloration, and thickening of nails. Sometimes, several joints are affected, while about one third of affected people also have spinal disease. Tendons and the site where tendons are attached to bones may also become inflamed, causing pain in the Achilles tendon, heels, and around the top of the thigh bone.

Q How is psoriatic arthritis treated?

Treatment for mild psoriatic arthritis may involve the use of splints to protect acutely inflamed joints. Physical therapy and exercises may be needed to help strengthen mildly inflamed joints. Your doctor may prescribe NSAIDs to combat the inflammation, and DMARDs and biologic agents (see pp90–93) to treat the causes of the disease.

Infective arthritis

Q Can arthritis be triggered by viruses, bacteria, and fungi?

Many important but relatively uncommon forms of arthritis are due to viral, bacterial, or fungal infections. They can occur by themselves or, sometimes, infective arthritis due to bacteria can complicate a preexisting inflammatory arthritis. Tuberculosis and lyme disease may also involve infective arthritis.

Q What happens when a virus causes arthritis?

Many forms of viral illness can cause an arthritis. This is usually of minor relevance, and aches and pains occur as part of feeling generally unwell. A viral arthritis tends to affect many joints and involves joint pain and stiffness rather than inflammation. It often occurs in the later stages of a viral illness and may come with a mild fever. Medical attention may be needed to prevent the joint from becoming permanently stiff (see box, p55).

Q What happens when an acute bacterial infection causes septic arthritis?

Acute bacterial infection tends to cause arthritis in one or more joints, which become hot, swollen, and red. Fever is a common occurrence. A sudden septic arthritis can affect a joint, with a high fever. People with preexisting arthritis are at a higher risk.

Q What is reactive arthritis?

Reactive arthritis is different to infective (septic) arthritis. It is inflammation of a joint caused by the immune system's response to a bacterial infection elsewhere in the body. It can be accompanied by rashes on hands or feet, diarrhea, conjunctivitis, mouth ulcers, and inflammation of the genital tract. Reactive arthritis usually lasts for 6 months or less, and long-term consequences are not common.

Q Can lyme disease cause arthritis?

Yes. This disease was first found in people from Old Lyme, Connecticut. The cause is a bacterium (*Borrelia burgdorferi*), transmitted from a bite of an infected tick. Initial symptoms are fever, fatigue, muscle pain, and a rash. After some months, many infected people develop arthritis, mainly in the large joints such as the knee.

Q Can tuberculosis cause arthritis?

Yes. Chronic infections such as tuberculosis can cause arthritis. About 1 in 100 people with tuberculosis develop an associated arthritis. It particularly involves the spine, hips, knees, wrists, or ankles. Symptoms include low-grade fever, increased sweating, fever at night, reduced joint mobility, and some swelling and tenderness of the joints.

TREATING INFECTIVE ARTHRITIS

Infective (septic) arthritis falls into several categories, according to whether the infection is caused by viruses, bacteria, or specific forms of infective agents. Accordingly, the treatment depends on the category.

Viral arthritis: needs only symptomatic treatment with rest, analgesics, and anti-inflammatory drugs; physical approaches such as hot/cold treatment or physical therapy may also help.

Infective arthritis due to bacteria: needs antibiotics, but the type and duration of treatment depend on the circumstances. In general terms, some patients require 2 or 3 different antibiotics, which will need to be used for a long time (usually 4–6 weeks) to fully eradicate the condition.

Specific forms of infective arthritis: need specific treatments for the relevant intracellular organism (for example, tuberculosis) or unusual infective agents such as fungi.

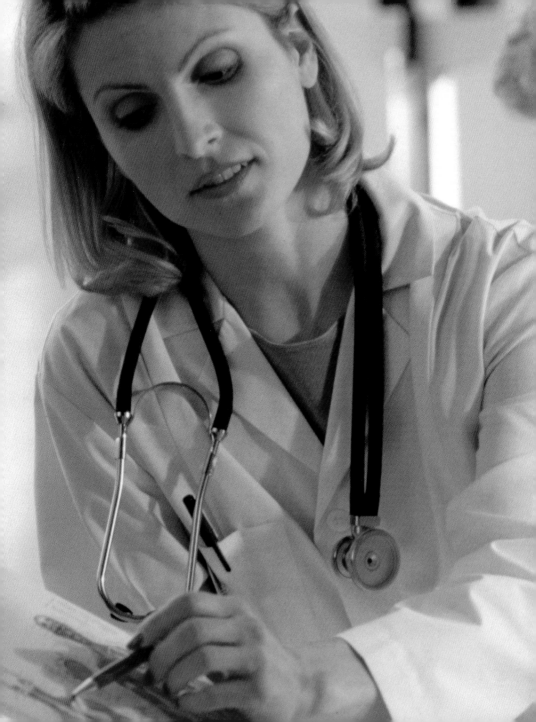

Diagnosis and healthcare

When a rheumatologist looks at
all your symptoms together,
a particular pattern emerges that
helps narrow down and identify
the type of arthritis affecting you.
You shouldn't feel helpless if you
are diagnosed with arthritis. Your
input in helping to manage your
own arthritis will always
be welcomed and encouraged
by your healthcare team.

Diagnosis

Q How can I make the most of my appointment with the doctor?

Visiting the doctor's office or attending a hospital clinic can be daunting, especially if you have been recently diagnosed with arthritis. Taking a friend or relative with you may help your communications with your doctor go more smoothly. Be prepared for your appointment and come with a concise list of the important questions you want to ask or points you want to discuss. Ask for an explanation of any medical terms and, if you want more information, say so. If you run out of time to discuss everything you want, make another appointment.

Q How can I establish a good relationship with my doctor?

Communication is the key to successful healthcare. As a patient, you can expect to receive the information you need from your doctor. It is equally important that he or she, in return, receives information from you. Your personal knowledge of how arthritis—and its treatment—affects you is valuable. Don't hesitate to share your concerns and speak openly of your needs, symptoms, and feelings. Building up a working partnership with your doctor will boost your confidence and help you feel in control of your arthritis.

Q Will my doctor be able to tell me whether or not I have arthritis?

By listening to your description of the symptoms (the history) and looking at what is wrong (the examination), your doctor will have a good idea of whether or not you have arthritis. He or she may recommend that you see a rheumatologist and/or have an X-ray (see p59). Various imaging techniques can help confirm—or eliminate—a diagnosis of a particular type of arthritis.

Q What information does my medical history contain?

Your medical history should include: the history of your arthritis, general problems, current and previous treatments, details of past diseases, your personal and work situation, and any occurrence of arthritis in relatives.

Q How does the examination and assessment help the doctor formulate a diagnosis?

To the uninitiated, doctors seem to ask questions, do a physical examination, and then reach a conclusion. In practice, however, it's different. If your doctor does not have a fair idea of the likely diagnosis within a minute or two of talking to you, it will probably be difficult to reach a diagnosis later. Examination helps the doctor make the diagnosis and helps in the evaluation of the severity of the disease and can pinpoint problems with specific joints.

Q What do X-rays reveal about arthritis?

Plain radiographs (X-rays) have traditionally been used for imaging joints. They show joint damage and provide an assessment of its severity and progression. In arthritis, they may reveal loss of bone, shown by the presence of erosions next to the margins of joints—a characteristic of rheumatoid arthritis. X-rays also reveal bone growth, especially the presence of osteophytes (bony spurs), and show the loss of cartilage. Finally, they can help the doctor decide whether joint replacement surgery is needed.

Q What other imaging techniques can be used in the diagnosis of arthritis?

Imaging techniques, such as computerized tomography (CT), magnetic resonance imaging (MRI), ultrasound, isotope bone scans, and dual-energy X-ray absorptiometry (DXA), can provide a more enhanced image of bones and joints than X-rays. Some, particularly MRI and ultrasound, can show inflammation and soft-tissue swelling. In the next 10 years, these techniques will probably replace X-rays as the preferred method for imaging joints.

Q Can blood tests help confirm the diagnosis of a particular type of arthritis?

Your doctor will almost certainly recommend blood tests. An analysis of your blood can help to confirm a diagnosis or indicate the severity of the disease. The tests are never diagnostic in their own right. They are often used to assess the safety and effectiveness of treatment as well.

Q What do blood tests look for?

Blood tests can reveal specific chemicals that are markers of arthritis. Tests are frequently done to measure uric acid levels in the blood, which are usually, but not necessarily, high in people with gout. However, individuals with a high uric acid level usually show no evidence of gout. In fact, in an acute attack of gout, uric acid levels may be normal. Blood tests also identify specific autoantibodies—antibodies that react with specific proteins in your body. They are thought to be the by-products of a disturbed immune system—a common feature in rheumatoid arthritis and some connective tissue diseases. One such autoantibody is rheumatoid factor, which may play a role in rheumatoid arthritis.

Q I've been told I need an ESR test —what is this?

The erythrocyte sedimentation rate (ESR) assesses the way your body responds to a damaging situation, such as an infection or inflammation, by measuring how fast red blood cells (erythrocytes) in a blood sample settle when left to stand. The faster they settle, the higher the ESR, and the more inflammation. It is measured in millimeters per hour. Normally, it is less than 20, but is often 50–100mm/hour in active rheumatoid arthritis, with a small decrease in numbers of red cells and changes in specific blood proteins. The most frequently measured protein is the C-reactive protein. This is normally less than 5mg/liter in the blood and can be 50–100mg/liter in active arthritis.

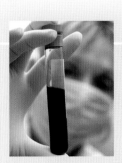

TESTS TO ANALYZE BLOOD

Blood contains many different substances, and blood tests can be used to analyze the cell content of the blood (red blood cells, white blood cells, and platelets), measure the erythrocyte sedimentation rate (ESR), and check for the levels of autoantibodies, such as rheumatoid factor and antinuclear antibodies.

BLOOD TEST	REASON FOR TEST
Blood count	To measure the level of hemoglobin. Low levels may indicate anemia—a blood disorder that might have a link to arthritis. High levels of white blood cells and platelets may indicate infection or inflammation.
Liver function	To measure levels of some enzymes to check if the liver is working properly and if it can deal with medicines such as methotrexate.
Kidney function	To measure the levels of waste products such as urea and creatine and certain dissolved salts in order to check that the kidneys are working properly.
Erythrocyte sedimentation rate (ESR)	To assess the body's response to a damaging situation, such as inflammation or infection.
Autoantibodies	To look for autoantibodies, such as rheumatoid factor and antinuclear antibodies. These may be able to help diagnose the different types of juvenile idiopathic arthritis.
C-reactive protein (CRP) levels	To measure the level of C-reactive protein—a type of protein produced by the liver when there is acute inflammation.

Q A blood test has revealed that I have rheumatoid factor. Does this mean I have, or will develop, rheumatoid arthritis?

Not necessarily. Rheumatoid factor is an autoantibody that can be detected by blood tests. It reacts with proteins that are released by the immune system. It is detected in about two-thirds of people with rheumatoid arthritis. However, its presence in the blood does not necessarily confirm rheumatoid arthritis because it can be associated with other diseases as well. The test for rheumatoid factor is only useful as a diagnostic test when considered with other tests.

Q The results of a blood test show that I have antinuclear antibodies—what are these?

Antinuclear antibodies are antibodies that react with components of the normal cell nucleus. They are characteristic of lupus, but also occur in most other connective tissue diseases, rheumatoid arthritis, and other generalized chronic inflammatory conditions. They are a family of different autoantibodies rather than a single and distinct autoantibody, and as a result they are very nonspecific. Nevertheless, it is usual for people with lupus to have some detectable antinuclear antibodies in their blood.

Q Will I need an operation such as an arthroscopy to see if my joint is affected by arthritis?

It may be necessary if your doctor thinks it would help examine a joint very thoroughly. An arthroscope is a small, flexible fiberoptic scope that can be inserted through a small incision in the skin to look inside large joints, such as the knee, and smaller joints, such as the wrist. For example, arthroscopy of the knee can distinguish between problems that are due to meniscus damage (torn knee cartilage) and problems resulting from arthritis. Arthroscopes can also be used to obtain a biopsy of the synovial tissue as a way of checking for infections, crystals, and cells.

Your healthcare team

Q Will my doctor continue to play an important role in helping me manage my arthritis?

Your doctor is your partner in caring for your arthritis and will be your primary point of contact for any long-term care. Many different health professionals may be involved in the diagnosis and treatment of your arthritis. Some you may see only once, others more frequently, or on an ongoing basis, depending on the type and severity of your arthritis. Nevertheless, your doctor will always help you manage your arthritis and can refer you to suitable specialists. If you have any concerns or questions about some aspect of your treatment, discuss these with your doctor.

Q Do I need to see a rheumatologist on a regular basis?

This depends on the nature of your arthritis and its severity. For example, your doctor may refer you to a rheumatologist if you have severe osteoarthritis or an inflammatory disorder, such as rheumatoid arthritis. Rheumatologists are doctors with specialist training in arthritis and other diseases that affect the joints. Your rheumatologist can interpret your tests (and may suggest more), discuss your treatment, prescribe drugs, or refer you for surgery, if it is required.

Q My doctor has referred me to an orthopedic surgeon—what do these specialists do?

Orthopedic doctors and surgeons specialize in treating muscle and bone disorders, as well as problems with the body's joints, tendons, and ligaments. Orthopedic surgeons perform joint replacement surgery, back surgery, and arthroscopic surgery (see pp94–113); some surgeons may even specialize in particular joints, such as the feet and ankles.

Playing an active role in managing your arthritis

Today, there are more treatment options available to you than ever before, from drugs and surgery to self-help measures and counseling. But no longer do you have to be a mere recipient of treatment.

GET THE BEST FROM YOUR TREATMENT

Try to take an active role in your arthritis management plan by learning about the treatment options and what you can expect from them. Being informed allows you to be more involved in decisions and able to communicate with your healthcare team.

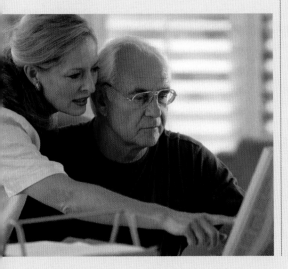

Management of arthritis differs from person to person, according to the severity of the condition and factors, such as how individuals tolerate certain drugs. What suits one person may not work as well with another—so make sure that your health professionals are aware of your personal needs and concerns. The more a doctor knows about you and your lifestyle, the more precisely the treatment can be tailored to your particular requirements.

Keep your doctor up to date with aspects that affect your quality of life. For example, your medication may cause unacceptable side effects or your exercise program may prove too strenuous. Prompt communication allows you and your doctor to prevent small problems from turning into major ones. You should also report the news of any improvements.

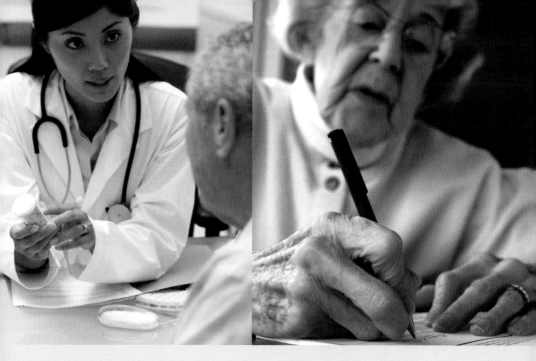

BE PROACTIVE

- Keep a diary to monitor your progress and the effects of any treatment. It will provide a handy record to discuss with your health professionals.
- If you are not satisfied with your healthcare, tell your doctor—this will not cause offence.
- Don't be afraid to suggest alternative treatments to your doctor, but be guided by his or her advice.
- When talking to your health professionals, be honest about how arthritis affects your personal life and emotional well-being.

BE CONSIDERATE

Your relationship with the healthcare professionals in your team will benefit if your attitude is helpful and your expectations are reasonable.

- Always try to arrive on time for an appointment; if you have to cancel, tell the doctor's office as soon as you can.
- If you are on refillable prescriptions, request a new prescription before you run out of pills. In some cases, pharmacies are willing to speak to doctors to refill a prescription medication rather than requiring you to present the actual signed prescription form from your doctor.

Q What do physical therapists do and can they visit me at home?

A physical therapist is a specialist in physical treatments that help restore movement and function in the body. He or she may use a range of methods, from massage and manipulation to the use of heat and hydrotherapy.
A physical therapist will first ask you about your condition and examine you, and then may suggest an appropriate course of treatment, which may require further sessions. Your physical therapist may also be able to visit you in your own home.

Q Can I make an appointment to see an occupational therapist whenever I need to?

Possibly. If your arthritis causes practical problems at home or at work, then an occupational therapist is the best person to turn to for help (see p119). Ask your doctor to refer you or approach the social services department directly.

Q Will I need to receive care from a nurse or nurse practitioner?

Nurses at your health center or at your doctor's office organize blood tests and provide advice on medication, among their many other roles. Nurse practitioners are highly experienced nurses who have received extra training in a state-approved training program, which allows them to take on certain roles traditionally carried out only by doctors.

Q If I need to change my diet do I need to see a dietitian or a nutritionist?

Either a dietician or a nutritionist would be able to help you. If you need to lose weight, your doctor may refer you to a dietitian for advice on what foods are best for you to eat. Dietitians must follow an established training program and be registered before they can practice. Nutritionists have a very similar role, but while they may also have undergone training, they are not required to be registered.

Q Can I see a counselor if I am struggling to come to terms with having arthritis?

Yes, talking to a counselor would help you through a difficult period. All doctors agree that pain is a complex and little understood process and many people believe there is a strong link between the mind and body. By talking things through with a professional counselor, you may make a very real difference to the level of pain and discomfort you experience. If you consult a counselor privately, make sure that he or she is either registered with an organization such as American Association of Psychotherapists or is a licensed marriage and family counselor.

Q Is it a good idea to join a support group?

Joining a support group is a good way of staying updated on new treatments, learning tips on coping with your condition and its symptoms, and getting in touch with others who share your experiences or problems. Look for groups that focus on your kind of arthritis. There are support groups for caregivers as well as for people with arthritis. Most groups provide helplines or free internet information. Find out about support groups and self-management programs on the Arthritis Foundation website (see Useful addresses, p184).

Q If I have chronic pain, is it worth going to a pain clinic?

Yes, especially if your pain is proving difficult to manage. Pain clinics typically employ a range of professionals, from nurses and doctors to complementary practitioners, such as acupuncturists, and others who use a variety of methods, such as drug injections and hydrotherapy, to control and relieve pain. Your own nurse or nurse practitioner will be able to locate the nearest pain clinic for you, or you can visit the Arthritis Foundation website (see Useful addresses, p184).

Q Is it unwise to buy drugs directly from websites?

Many regulatory organizations, as well as professional organizations such as the American Medical Association, warn against buying drugs online. Although there are genuine online pharmacies, many are entirely unregulated so the drugs they offer may not be reliable and vital patient information may be missing. You should only buy medicines from regular pharmacies and on your doctor's advice. Whether you're buying drugs or seeking information, always check the provider's credentials with the relevant organization. Be wary of advice that contradicts the information given by your doctor.

Q Is it OK to rely on over-the-counter medicines?

Yes, as long as you have been given a diagnosis and your doctor is aware that you are taking them. Taking calcium and vitamin D is useful in helping to prevent osteoporosis in at-risk groups. Whenever you buy an over-the-counter drug, read the accompanying information carefully and take the correct dosage as some drugs can be dangerous if not taken properly or combined with prescription medicines. Taking over-the-counter medicines also gives you a measure of control, enabling you to become an active participant rather than a passive recipient in managing your condition.

Q What's the difference between generic and brand-name drugs?

All medicines have an approved, or generic, name. Acetaminophen and ibuprofen are examples of generic names. Generic drugs are usually cheaper than branded ones. Brands and generics usually contain different buffers, additives, and fillers but the active ingredients are the same. There are strict laws to ensure that both generic and brand-name drugs are equally effective and safe to use.

WHAT STEPS CAN I TAKE TO HELP MYSELF?

You may find that drugs or surgery alone are unable to keep your arthritis in check. Regardless of whether you need extra medical help, the following self-help strategies will make a difference and almost certainly improve your overall quality of life. They may even bring some relief from symptoms such as pain and inflammation.

- Make changes to your lifestyle— you may only need to make minor adjustments if you are affected mildly.

- Think positively about the condition that is affecting you.

- Exercise regularly (see p168) or practice exercise routines (see pp172–175).

- Learn the various techniques that can help you cope with the episodes of pain (see p136) and the stress you may feel (see p140).

- Teach yourself relaxation or meditation techniques that will help you stay calm when tension and anxiety start to build up within you.

- Eat a healthy diet with fresh fruit and vegetables (see pp146–156). Maintain a healthy weight (see pp160–161).

- Drink alcohol in moderation and don't smoke.

- Try complementary therapies, such as massage (see p76), but check with your doctor before beginning any herbal medicines (see pp72–73), which might interact with prescription medicines.

- Ask your family and friends for help with everyday tasks, such as shopping and household chores.

- Discover ways to cope with everyday problems (see pp121–123).

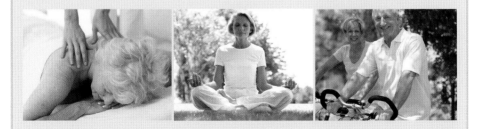

Complementary healthcare

Q **How can complementary therapies help my arthritis?**

When used wisely, complementary therapies may help relieve certain symptoms or contribute to your sense of well-being. Some may help you relax, reduce stress, or encourage sleep, which in turn may help relieve pain.

Q **What sort of complementary therapies could be helpful?**

Complementary therapies include natural remedies, such as herbs and homeopathy, bodywork therapies, such as massage and reflexology, and movement therapies, such as yoga and tai chi. Some, such as herbal medicine, are ancient while others are new. Therapies should complement, but not replace, your regular treatment.

Q **How can I find a qualified and reputable practitioner?**

With an almost equal proportion of highly trained and not-so-highly trained practitioners available, one needs to choose carefully. Many of the more established complementary therapies are self-regulated by their professional bodies. Practitioners who wish to be listed with a professional body must adhere to certain standards, such as completing a certified level of training. In return, the practitioner can be registered on an approved list. In addition, all complementary therapists must be licensed by the state where they want to practice, and the requirements vary from state to state.

Q **Can I locate a complementary practitioner online?**

You can access an approved list online, but remember that health advice on the Internet is hardly regulated. Do check the credentials of the websites you look at, be wary of advice that contradicts your doctor's, and be cautious of websites that sell services or products.

Q **If I visit a complementary therapist, should I tell my doctor?**

If you have heard that a specific therapy may be able to help your arthritis, the best step is to first talk to your doctor, who may be able to recommend an experienced practitioner in your locality. In fact, your doctor may even be the first to suggest a therapist as part of your treatment. If you are already trying a complementary therapy, be sure to keep your doctor or rheumatologist informed. They can tell you if a particular herb or supplement is safe to take at the same time as any existing medication; they will also know whether a therapy suits your level of overall health and mobility. It may help you to take notes of any changes a therapy brings to your health—good or bad—which you can then discuss with your doctor.

Q **Are there any herbal remedies that may help relieve inflammation and pain?**

Few herbs have been scientifically tested for their effect on the symptoms of arthritis, but there is evidence to suggest that some may help to relieve inflammation and pain. These include cat's claw, ginger, and turmeric (see pp72–73). You shouldn't take any of these, or any other herb, without first consulting your doctor and herbal medicine expert.

Q **Is it worth trying acupuncture?**

It may be, because acupuncture may be useful for many conditions, including the pain from osteoarthritis and fibromyalgia, as well as nausea, headache, depression, and back pain. However, evidence for its effectiveness is mixed and depends on the condition: there is strong evidence that it is effective for dental pain and nausea, promising evidence for fibromyalgia, but conflicting evidence for treating back pain and osteoarthritis. Acupuncture has been shown to facilitate the release of certain chemicals called endorphins in the brain that may ease pain.

Herbal medicines

Few traditional herbs have been tested for their effect on the symptoms of arthritis, but evidence suggests that some may help relieve inflammation and pain.

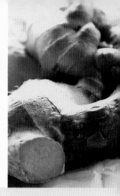

CAT'S CLAW

This vine (*Uncaria tomentosa*) grows in the Peruvian rainforest and has thorns shaped like cat's claws. The root bark is a traditional remedy for inflammation and has been used for boosting immunity, as well as for treating arthritic and gastrointestinal complaints. Some recent studies suggest it may be useful for treating osteoarthritis and rheumatoid arthritis. The recommended dosage is 500–1,000mg taken as capsules, 3 times a day. Medical herbalists often avoid using it with hormonal drugs, insulin, or vaccines because of potential interaction.

DEVIL'S CLAW

This shrub (*Harpagophytum procumbens*) grows in southern Africa and has hooked, clawlike seed pods. It contains a substance called harpagoside, which has been shown in two trials to reduce inflammation and pain. This herb has been traditionally used for pain and inflammation and is a popular remedy among people with rheumatoid arthritis. You can take it as a capsule, or as a tincture or tea. However, it may interfere with warfarin or drugs used for irregular heartbeats and diabetes. Check with your doctor first if you have gallstones or gastric or duodenal ulcers. Avoid devil's claw if you are pregnant or are taking NSAIDs (see p83).

CAYENNE

Also known as paprika, chili pepper, or red pepper, cayenne (*Capsicum frutescens*) is a traditional remedy for conditions, such as arthritic pain and stomach upsets. Its active ingredient, capsaicin, stimulates the release of endorphins, the body's natural pain relievers. Although there is little evidence of its effectiveness, many people with arthritis regularly rub capsaicin cream into their affected joints. You should avoid putting the cream on broken or irritated skin. Wash your hands thoroughly after use. Eating too much cayenne can be very dangerous because it affects your body temperature.

GINGER

The root of ginger (*Zingiber officinale*) is a traditional remedy for digestive disorders, such as nausea, and arthritic pain. One trial showed that ginger eased the pain of osteoarthritis. It may help relieve pain and inflammation because it seems to block the action of chemicals in the body, such as leukotrienes, that cause pain and swelling. Cook with ginger regularly but avoid it if you are taking blood-thinning drugs, such as warfarin, or if you have gallstones, diabetes, or heart problems —unless your doctor approves.

TURMERIC

A spice familiar to cooks, turmeric (*Curcuma longa*) has been used in traditional Chinese and Ayurvedic medicine to ease inflammation and pain in arthritis. Small studies suggest that it has an effect when used in combination with other supplements, but there is no scientific evidence that it works alone. High doses of turmeric may act as a blood-thinner and may also cause gastrointestinal upsets. You should avoid turmeric if you have gallstones.

BROMELAIN

Bromelain, a protein-digesting enzyme, is extracted from the pineapple plant (*Ananas comosus*). Several trials suggest it is anti-inflammatory and may help relieve pain in arthritis. The recommended dosage is 400–600mg of bromelain extract, 3 times a day. You should avoid taking bromelain supplements during pregnancy or while breast-feeding. It may interfere with blood-thinning drugs, such as warfarin, and large doses may cause stomach upsets.

BURDOCK

The root of burdock (*Arctium lappa*) has been used for many conditions, including arthritis. However, there is no convincing scientific evidence to suggest that it is effective. If you suffer from diabetes, always check with your doctor before taking it. Burdock may also affect birth control pills, hormone therapy (HT), and blood-thinning drugs, such as warfarin or heparin.

BOSWELLIA

This tree (*Boswellia thurifera*) produces the frankincense resin used in traditional Chinese and Ayurvedic medicine for arthritic pain relief. Some trials show it is effective in relieving inflammation in arthritis, especially when combined with an Indian herb called ashwagandha. However, there is little evidence to confirm that it is safe. The recommended dosage is 150mg of boswellia extract, taken 3 times a day.

Myth "Natural remedies are safe because they are not man-made"

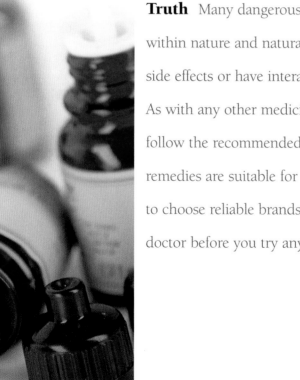

Truth Many dangerous substances are found within nature and natural remedies may still cause side effects or have interactions with other drugs. As with any other medicine, you should always follow the recommended dosage. Not all natural remedies are suitable for everyone, so it is vital to choose reliable brands and to speak to your doctor before you try any new remedy.

Q What homeopathic medicines help in arthritis?

A registered homeopath who is experienced in treating arthritis may recommend one of several medicines to relieve symptoms. Some evidence suggests that *Rhus toxicodendron* may help with morning stiffness that affects people with osteoarthritis. *Apis mellifica* may help the hot, swollen, and tender joints that are common in rheumatoid arthritis. Causticum may help people who have joints that seem to be very weather-sensitive.

Q What sort of benefits can I expect from movement therapies such as yoga, tai chi, Pilates, or Qi Gong?

Ensuring mobility is very important for people with arthritis (see p158). When joints are stiff or sore, it is often tempting to avoid using them, but this can lead to greater pain and disability. Movement therapies, such as yoga, tai chi, Pilates, Qi Gong, and the Alexander technique teach new ways of holding, stretching, and moving your body. These changes will bring about improvements to your posture that might not only ease symptoms, but also lead to an overall sensation of well-being.

Q Is it worth trying the Alexander technique to help with my posture?

Perhaps it is. The Alexander technique is based on the idea that the head, neck, and spine play a crucial role in the overall flexibility and health of the body. Over the years, you have probably developed awkward ways of sitting, standing, and moving. You unconsciously tense up with anxiety or stress and adopt poor postures that affect the way you move your body. Teachers who practice this technique work with people on a one-to-one basis to show them how to correct postural problems and use the body in a more "natural" way. The technique has been beneficial for people with respiratory problems and back pain, and works on the body's autonomic nervous system to help relieve stress and anxiety.

Q Would a massage be good for my arthritic symptoms?

A massage may help you relax and relieve the stress of arthritis. Modern massage, also known as Swedish massage, was developed in the 19th century by a Swede called Per Henrik Ling. There are many different kinds of massage techniques now that are gentler than Ling's vigorous methods. There are various soft-tissue massage techniques (see soft-tissue massage, p77), some of which may also use aromatherapy oils. Massage is used for a wide range of conditions, from back pain and fibromyalgia to irritable bowel syndrome, headaches, and general stress relief, and the evidence to support its use is relatively good. However, as with any touch therapy, you must take extra care when joints are inflamed. Check with your doctor or rheumatologist whether massage is right for you.

Q Will manipulation and bodywork practices help to relieve my pain or restore any lost function in my joints?

They might. Manipulation and bodywork practices, such as massage, chiropractic, and osteopathy, are among the more respected and trustworthy of the complementary therapies. In experienced hands, they aim to ease restrictions, alleviate pain, and restore loss of function. At the core, they seek to rebalance the body's equilibrium and reestablish the integrated nature of the musculoskeletal system. It is still important to have a trusted therapist and to take care when joints are inflamed.

Q Are there any other bodywork or manipulation therapies that may help relieve my symptoms?

Yes, although there's very little conclusive evidence to prove they actually work. Clinical aromatherapy is said to increase vitality, improve general well-being, and restore health. The essential oils of aromatherapy may help with various ailments, such as anxiety and insomnia. Reflexology, as with any massage, helps you relax and may bring some relief from stress.

SOFT-TISSUE MASSAGE

Massage, in its various forms, may relieve arthritic symptoms such as pain, stiffness, tension, and immobility. It increases blood flow to the muscles to reduce tension, thereby relieving pain and encouraging mobility. However, you should avoid massage if you have a flare-up of symptoms.

THERAPY	WHAT DOES IT INVOLVE?	HOW MIGHT IT HELP?
Swedish massage	Kneading (petrissage) or rhythmic stroking (effleurage) of muscles and soft tissues; may include oils or electrical stimulation devices.	Reduces general stiffness and releases tension. Benefits osteoarthritis, rheumatoid arthritis, and fibromyalgia.
Chair massage	Manipulation in a specially designed chair that bends your body to improve the practitioner's access to your tense joints.	Neck and back joint pain, fibromyalgia, and arthritic pain—so long as you can sit comfortably in the chair.
Myofascial release	Slow, gentle manipulation of your fascia—the thin tissues surrounding muscles—to stretch your tense tissues and relieve pain and stress.	Fibromyalgia and general stress relief associated with any chronic illness.
Deep-tissue massage	Releases tension in deeper layers of soft tissue, with manipulation across the grain of your muscle; it may also break up scar tissue within the soft tissues.	General arthritis. It is especially good for back pain that is associated with arthritis.

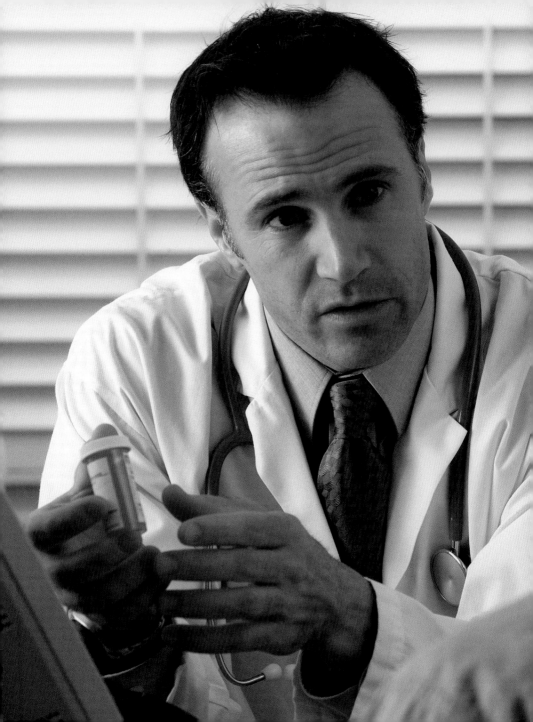

Drug treatments

Over the last few decades, pharmacologists have increasingly tried to match specific drug treatments to particular diseases. They no longer seek to combat all the different types of arthritis and related musculoskeletal disorders with one magic formula. In most cases of arthritis, drug treatment is used in combination with other methods, such as physical therapy.

Taking medication

Q **What happens when I start medication for arthritis?**

Most people who have arthritis need to start taking medication at some stage of the disease. Usually, the treatment proceeds in a step-wise fashion, moving from the simple to the more complicated drugs, which may be given either alone or in combination, depending on the severity of your disease. Your doctor may prescribe analgesics and nonsteroidal anti-inflammatory drugs (NSAIDs) in the early stages of many types of arthritis and then refer you to a rheumatologist, who can prescribe drugs that may be more potent.

Q **Are there any general rules for taking drugs safely?**

Before you take any drug, make sure you know all about it and how it is expected to help. Find out all the details about its dosage—how much you need to take, how often you need to take it, and at what time of the day. Draw up a timetable to help to remember everything. Be aware of any potential interactions with other drugs or with any herbs, supplements, or natural remedies you may be taking.

Q **Can I buy any anti-arthritic drugs over the counter at a pharmacy?**

You can buy a small number of anti-arthritic drugs over the counter after taking advice from the pharmacist who sells them. However, do not totally rely on the pharmacist to make a balanced decision for you. Always ask your doctor about the pros and cons—you may find the chances of a risky interaction outweigh the benefits of a drug. Carefully read the given information and take the correct dosage.

Should I believe what I read about medications on the Internet?

Not necessarily. Many people turn to the Internet and look online for information about health. Much of it is accurate, updated, and useful, but some websites are unreliable. Remember, there is often little or no regulation of health information on the Internet.

How will I know what the side effects of my prescribed drug will be?

Your doctor should be able to present both the advantages and disadvantages of a particular drug treatment, allowing you to make your own informed decision. It is only natural you should be concerned about the side effects of your medications. But, at the same time, don't forget the benefits you are likely to receive from the drug.

How can I be sure there will be no interactions between the anti-arthritic drug and any other medication I might be taking?

Your doctor has access to an up-to-date list of possible drug interactions and so will be able to check this list against other drugs you might be taking and draw your attention to the most serious interactions. Doctors who prescribe drugs such as anticoagulants, which are notorious for interaction, will also provide you with whatever warnings you need.

Can I take drugs by applying them to the skin around affected joints?

NSAIDs, analgesics, and homeopathic remedies are usually available as a cream or paste for applying to the skin around your affected joints. These topical agents are absorbed through the skin more slowly than when taken orally. Therefore, side effects are reduced but by no means completely avoided. You can also apply capsaicin. The manufacturers of capsaicin point out that its only side effect is pain at the point of application, but people soon acclimatize to this, especially if very small amounts are applied.

Myth "Rubbing topical agents directly on to the skin relieves pain more quickly"

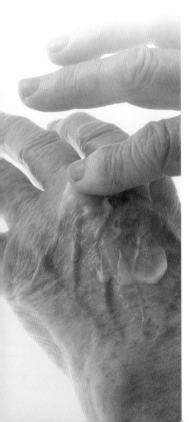

Truth Topical agents are absorbed more slowly than when taken orally and there is little evidence that they remain in the joint for a significant period of time before they are dispersed by the blood's circulation. If they linger in the tissues adjacent to the joint, they may provide some local benefit, though they may also work partly by suggestion. Any benefit is often short term. Some people enjoy applying cream to the affected area because they feel that they are actively doing something to help.

Analgesics and NSAIDs

Q What are analgesics good for?

Analgesics are drugs that help relieve the mild to moderate pain of several types of arthritis. There are 2 main types—the opioids and the nonpioids. Opioids, including codeine and hydrocodone, are strong analgesics with effects similar to drugs derived from opium, such as morphine. Nonopioids include tramadol, acetaminophen, and NSAIDs, such as aspirin and ibuprofen.

Q Which analgesics can I buy over the counter?

Acetaminophen is the simplest analgesic commonly available over the counter. Aspirin, naproxen, ketoprofen, and ibuprofen are also commonly available.

Q Do analgesics have any side effects?

Acetaminophen, which is different from aspirin, can safely be taken in a dose of 500mg up to 8 times a day (normally as 2 tablets 4 times a day or as required) without any major side effects. However, avoid higher doses, which can cause liver damage, and refrain from alcohol use. Aspirin and other NSAIDs may cause gastrointestinal problems. In fact, aspirin is hardly ever used in arthritis since the doses required for pain relief are very high and the side effects exceed those from ibuprofen and the other NSAIDs.

Q If acetaminophen doesn't help with my pain, do I need a prescription for a more powerful analgesic?

Acetaminophen alone may relieve the pain of arthritis. If it fails to do so, and your doctor confirms that you have osteoarthritis, you can move to more potent medications, such as tramadol or tramadol with acetaminophen. If neither of these treatments help, your doctor may consider more potent analgesics, such as propoxyphene or codeine.

Q I've been relying on one analgesic for years but now I hear that it has been withdrawn. Does this mean I can't use it anymore?

Drugs remain under constant review by licensing agencies in most countries (in the US, by the Food and Drug Administration), and pharmaceutical companies continue to examine data accumulated through clinical trials and other medical research. For example, the manufacturer of the COX-2 inhibitor rofecoxib took it off the market in 2004 due to safety concerns—a study had indicated that there was an increased risk of heart disease and strokes for those who took the drug for chronic arthritis pain.

Q What are NSAIDs good for?

NSAIDs are widely prescribed because they help people with many different types of arthritis, particularly those with an inflammatory component and those in which the joints are swollen, stiff, and sometimes a little hot, rather than just painful. They are called non-steroidal because they do not contain corticosteroids, which can have powerful side effects. In early arthritis, you will normally be prescribed NSAIDs, such as naproxen, ketoprofen, indomethacin, and diclofenac, after you have tried analgesics.

Q Which NSAIDs can I buy over the counter at a pharmacy?

Three NSAIDs—ibuprofen, naproxen, and ketoprofen—is available over the counter and these are in lower doses than that normally prescribed for arthritis by rheumatologists and other doctors.

Q Do NSAIDs have any side effects?

NSAIDs have more side effects than analgesics such as acetaminophen, although people who need them find them extremely effective. Side effects of NSAIDs include gastrointestinal irritation, a slight but reversible change in kidney function, and a slightly increased risk of stroke and heart attack.

Q Could I avoid the gastric side effects of NSAIDs by taking them as a suppository?

No, not really. Many gastric side effects actually result from the breakdown products of the drugs circulating in the blood rather than direct irritation of the stomach. Using suppositories as a route of delivery reduces the risk only slightly.

CHOOSING THE RIGHT NSAID

There are up to 15 or 20 NSAIDs marketed at present. It is important to consult a doctor before you decide which NSAID to take to manage your pain cycle. You and your doctor may wish to consider the following factors when choosing the best NSAID for you:

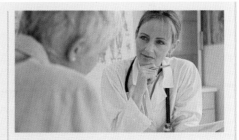

- The family to which an NSAID belongs has some bearing on the side effects you are likely to experience, such as gastrointestinal irritation.

- The length of time an NSAID lasts when a single pill is taken is important. This is the drug's half-life. Some pills have a short half-life and need to be taken 4 or 5 times a day; others need to be taken just once a day.

- The way an NSAID works on the inflammation process may be important. Usually, an NSAID blocks the action of a particular chemical in the body, known as an inflammatory mediator.

COST CONCERNS: If the cost of a drug is a concern, you are likely to be prescribed older generic NSAIDs. The choice is usually one of the following three: short-acting drugs, such as ibuprofen and ketoprofen, that need to be taken 4 or more times a day; drugs such as diclofenac and naproxen that need to be taken 2 or 3 times a day; and drugs such as piroxicam that need to be taken only once a day. If these medications don't suit and frequent dosing is inconvenient, slow-release preparations of the shorter-acting drugs are also available.

Q Are there any new NSAIDs that don't cause gastrointestinal problems?

NSAIDs cause stomach problems because they block the action of a protective enzyme called COX-1. For this reason, they are sometimes called COX-1 inhibitors. A relatively new type of NSAID is known as a COX-2 inhibitor; an example is celecoxib. COX-2 inhibitors may be more efficaceous in protecting the gastrointestinal tract when compared to the older drugs.

Q Are there any risks in taking COX-2 inhibitors?

Experience obtained from several years of prescribing COX-2 inhibitors indicated that they could, along with the older NSAIDs, predispose people to heart and circulatory disorders. However, this is rare and many rheumatologists feel that if everyone taking COX-2 inhibitors returned to the earlier medicines that lead to gastric damage, the overall death rate from gastrointestinal effects would far exceed the death rate from the cardiovascular side effects of COX-2 inhibitors. It has been suggested that the risk of even a mild stroke or heart attack is so small that such a cardiovascular event will only occur roughly once every 400 patient years of treatment and perhaps even less often.

Q Do the concerns about COX-2 inhibitors mean they are no longer available?

The COX-2 inhibitors rofecoxib and valdecoxib were withdrawn in 2004 and 2005 respectively; celecoxib is still being sold. Following a review in 2005 by the FDA (Food and Drug Administration), doctors were advised to prescribe the lowest effective dose for the shortest duration possible for any NSAID. You should discuss the risks with your doctor. A family history of heart disease or stroke do not restrict the use of a COX-2 inhibitor, but if you once had either condition, seek medical advice.

Corticosteroids

Q Will corticosteroids help my arthritis?

Steroid use in early rheumatoid arthritis remains controversial. There is stronger reason to use steroids when the disease is accompanied by inflammation of the arteries. For some conditions, such as polymyalgia rheumatica (see p42) and giant cell arteritis, steroids are very effective.

Q Do corticosteroids have any side effects?

Corticosteroids are very effective in suppressing inflammation but they cause a wide range of side effects that detract significantly from their use. These include suppression of adrenal glands, high blood pressure, peptic ulcers, diabetes, glaucoma, cataracts, and osteoporosis. Corticosteroid use also causes the skin to become fragile, and wounds to heal more slowly.

Q Can I have an injection of corticosteroids into my arthritic joint?

Drugs injected directly into the affected joint—a technique called intra-articular injections—may be successful for many types of arthritis. The drug normally given is a steroid, which is helpful when the inflammatory arthritis occurs at a single joint. Your doctor can reduce the risks of the side effects by choosing a relatively insoluble steroid, which can remain in the joint for a longer peroid of time.

Q Will injections of lubricants help my osteoarthritis?

A wide variety of lubricants, such as hyaluronic acid, have been developed for use in intra-articular injection. These lubricants are more expensive than steroids but their use may be more effective if your condition does not involve inflammation. Lubricants tend to be used to alleviate the symptoms of osteoarthritis for a short period of time.

Drug treatment of osteoarthritis

Q Can osteoarthritis be cured with drugs?

No drugs affect the development of osteoarthritis once it has started. All you can expect is that analgesics will ease your pain and stiffness. Your doctor can prescribe strong painkillers, either singly or in combination, and NSAIDs to control any inflammation that occurs.

Q If I start treatment early can I prevent my osteoarthritis from getting worse?

Osteoarthritis progresses gradually so it is difficult to know whether early intervention has had an effect. It often runs in a family and it is doubtful if early treatment would eliminate this genetic risk. Gentle exercise and weight control may be the best bet for prevention. Analgesics or NSAIDs are unlikely to prevent disease progression although glucosamine and chondroitin might, particularly at the knee.

Q Is it better to take drugs throughout the day or when I know I'll need them?

If the pain occurs only when you exercise, perhaps at a predictable time of day, it is better to take a drug with a short half-life (see p85) just before you need it, rather than dosing yourself throughout the day.

Q What does the future hold for the treatment of osteoarthritis?

Much research is focused on finding drugs that modify the disease process rather than just mask its symptoms. Some claim that substances such as glucosamine, chondroitin sulfate, and vitamins do this, but the evidence is weak. Biologic agents recently introduced for rheumatoid arthritis might block the production of interleukins, which may be involved in osteoarthritis.

NSAID TREATMENT FOR OSTEOARTHRITIS

Weight-bearing joints such as the hip are particularly prone to the cartilage damage that is a feature of osteoarthritis. NSAIDs are commonly used to treat the pain and stiffness that accompanies the condition by reducing the inflammation in the joint. NSAIDs do not cure the disease, nor do they halt its progress. Damage to the cartilage and bone tissue is followed by a response from the body's immune system and the release of chemicals called prostaglandins, which cause inflammation and pain. By stopping the production of these prostaglandins, NSAIDs are able to reduce the inflammation in the joint and reduce the pain.

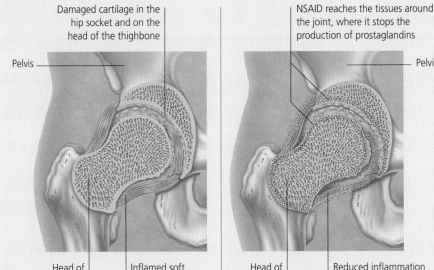

Damaged cartilage in the hip socket and on the head of the thighbone

NSAID reaches the tissues around the joint, where it stops the production of prostaglandins

Pelvis

Pelvis

Head of thighbone

Inflamed soft tissue surrounding the joint

Head of thighbone

Reduced inflammation in the soft tissues surrounding the joint

BEFORE TREATMENT *The cartilage in an osteoarthritic hip is damaged and the joint tissue is inflamed.*

AFTER TREATMENT *NSAID treatment reduces inflammation and so helps to relieve pain, but only as long as the drug is administered.*

Drug treatment of rheumatoid arthritis

Q Can rheumatoid arthritis be cured with drugs?

Possibly not. Various analgesics help relieve the pain and NSAIDs can combat the inflammation. An increasing number of drugs (DMARDs and biologic agents) help slow down the progress of the disease once it has started.

Q If I start the treatment early can I prevent rheumatoid arthritis from getting worse?

Yes, it is possible. Rheumatoid arthritis is an inflammatory condition that involves the joint lining and tendons and tendon sheaths around the joint. As it progresses, it can affect other body parts, such as the eyes, heart, lungs, skin, and blood vessels. Iwwf the inflammation is detected early and treated aggressively with DMARDs within the first few months, it may not develop into a severe condition.

Q Can corticosteroids reduce the inflammation?

Yes, they can be very effective. Prednisone is frequently prescribed for rheumatoid arthritis. Steroids can also be injected directly into inflamed joints, but their side effects require doctors to be careful about the dosage and duration. Although you will be monitored, it is important that you don't suddenly change or stop your medication.

Q If NSAIDs or corticosteroids fail, will I be given the disease-modifying antirheumatic drugs (DMARDs)?

Probably, because the powerful DMARDs can tackle the disease process of rheumatoid arthritis. They may not be able to stop it in its tracks, but can usually slow it down. Various tried and tested, and relatively inexpensive, DMARDs are available (see pp92-93), and may be used alone or in combination.

Q How often do I need to take DMARDs and for how long?

DMARDs act slowly, so you might not feel their effect for several weeks or months. Due to their side effects, and because different people respond to individual DMARDs in different ways, your rheumatologist will determine how long you need to take them.

Q If individual DMARDs fail, will my rheumatologist try a combination of them or will I be prescribed the new biologic agents?

Depending on your needs, you might receive either. When prescribing a course of combined drugs, a rheumatologist usually reviews the many DMARDs in turn, then proposes a specific combination on the basis of each person's disposition. One such combination uses sulfasalazine, methotrexate, and hydroxychloroquine. Alternatively, you may be given a biologic agent (see p93), which is injected.

Q Will I be prescribed biologic agents before DMARDs?

Perhaps. It's possible that biologic agents will be increasingly used early in the disease. Because of their considerable expense, they were mostly used later, after all other DMARDs had been tried. However, as rheumatologists are prescribing them with increasing confidence and registries show no unexpected or serious side effects, biologic agents are being used at an ever earlier stage. However, to supplant existing DMARDs right at the beginning, we still need evidence that proves biologics to be significantly better and to have equal safety.

Q My husband and I are hoping to start a family. Will the DMARDs I'm taking affect the baby?

Yes, DMARDs may cause problems, especially in the first 3 months of pregnancy. As a general rule, you may need to stop them for 3 to 6 months before conceiving. Ask your doctor about the risks before becoming pregnant. You may need an alternative regime to help you cope with your symptoms until you conceive. Some people find that pregnancy improves their rheumatoid arthritis.

Common DMARDs

A wide variety of DMARDs, including the biologic agents, may be prescribed in the treatment of rheumatoid arthritis. The following list is organized into the most commonly prescribed, starting with methotrexate:

METHOTREXATE

Developed as a potent anticancer drug, methotrexate was found to be effective for psoriasis and psoriatic arthritis and, later, for the closely related rheumatoid arthritis. Since the start of the 1990s, most rheumatologists have regarded it as the most effective treatment for rheumatoid arthritis. Dosage is calculated according to one's needs, but it normally averages 20mg a week. Some prefer intramuscular injection, which is often tried if the pills fail to work. Regular blood tests monitor the accumulation of methotrexate in the bone marrow and liver, and folic acid is given to offset side effects.

LEFLUNOMIDE

Introduced in the mid-1990s, this drug is specifically designed for treating rheumatoid arthritis. It blocks one pathway in cell multiplication, arresting the spread of the disease. In many cases, it is a second choice after methotrexate. Side effects may include elevated blood pressure, increased susceptibility to infection, and weight loss.

SULFASALAZINE

Developed for use in rheumatoid arthritis almost 50 years ago, this drug was used to treat ulcerative colitis and Crohn's disease before being reevaluated in the 1980s. Sulfasalazine is widely used and, although it shares some side effects with methotrexate (such as damage to the bone marrow and liver, and skin rash), they are less severe. Regular blood checks are required.

HYDROXYCHLOROQUINE

An antimalarial drug, hydroxychloroquine, was found by chance to improve the symptoms of rheumatoid arthritis. Regular eye examinations are needed to detect a deterioration in vision, although this is a very rare side effect. Otherwise, it is relatively safe although of modest efficacy.

AZATHIOPRINE

This prototype of a group of drugs developed against cancer prevents multiplication of cells. Since rheumatoid arthritis is essentially a disease in which the synovium proliferates, low doses may be effective. It has largely been replaced by methotrexate. Regular blood checks monitor any damage to the bone marrow. Other side effects are skin rash and liver damage.

CYCLOSPORIN

Developed from a fungus to prevent rejection of kidney transplants, cyclosporin has some action on rheumatoid arthritis. Arguably, much less effective than methotrexate or some other drugs, it is now used less frequently. Regular monitoring of side effects (raised blood pressure and impairment of kidney function) is needed.

INJECTABLE GOLD

Introduced to treat tuberculosis, gold injections were found to stabilize rheumatoid arthritis. Regular blood checks monitor any suppression of the bone marrow. Other side effects include skin rash and kidney damage. Because of this, gold shots are rarely used today. An oral gold preparation, auranofin, is available but can cause diarrhea, which limits its use.

BIOLOGIC AGENTS

In the 1990s, scientists found that rheumatoid arthritis is switched on in the body by a chemical messenger called a cytokine, which is known as TNF-alpha.

They discovered that another cytokine, known as IL-1, plays a secondary role in triggering the disease. Medical researchers have since developed a group of drugs named biologic agents to block and thereby neutralize these cytokines. There are 6 such biologic agents available: infliximab, etanercept, and adaminulab all block the action of TNF-alpha; anakinra blocks IL-1; abatacept inhibits T-cell function; and rifuximab selectively depletes B-cells.

The next 2–3 years are likely to see the licensing of a number of further TNF-alpha blockers, a further IL-1 blocker and one or more blockers of a third cytokine, IL-6. All these drugs are currently under trial, most showing some promise.

There is also at least one new biologic approach. Most biologic agents ultimately act on white blood cells known as T cells. However, another drug, called rituximab, actually acts against white blood cells known as B cells. Rituximab was developed to treat certain cancers (mainly lymphomas), but is showing some promise for rheumatoid arthritis as well. Because it is already licensed for another indication, an increasing number of rheumatologists are using it on a "orphan drug" basis when the T-cell biologic agents have failed—and sometimes before. There is reason to believe that rituximab will be licensed formally for rheumatoid arthritis.

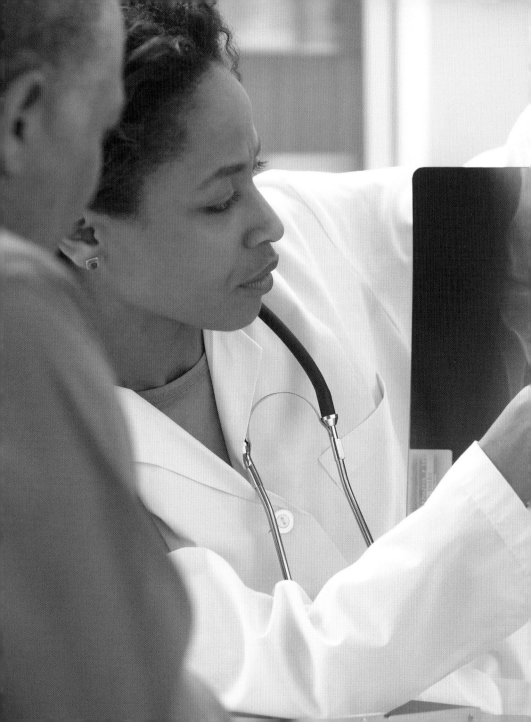

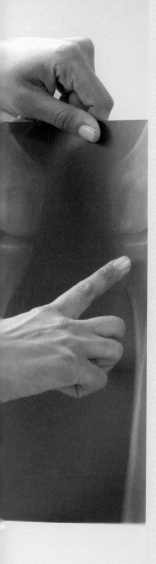

Surgical treatments

Modern surgical treatments
that focus on specific joints are
refined, relatively safe, and usually
successful. In fact, joint replacement
surgery, particularly of the hip, has
become one of the most effective
surgical treatments in medicine.
Surgeons now place considerable
emphasis on preparing people prior
to their operation, while
other healthcare professionals focus
on improving recovery
and rehabilitation.

Surgical options

Q **How bad does my pain have to be before I become eligible for surgery?**

If one of your joints is damaged to the point where the pain cannot be controlled with drugs or the joint can barely move, then surgery may be the only answer. No matter which type of arthritis you have, you might need surgery if you continue to feel pain in one of your joints, despite the best efforts of other treatments. You and your surgeon need to weigh risks and benefits before making a decision about surgery. Advice from other health professionals and your family may also be needed.

Q **Who performs surgery for arthritis?**

Surgery for arthritis, and replacing joints in particular, is a highly specialized branch of orthopedic surgery. It has evolved from setting fractures in plaster to treating skeletal deformities, replacing joints, and dealing with complex trauma. Many surgeons specialize solely in replacing joints, concentrating on the hip, knee, or shoulder. Training can take a long time—often 10 years or more after qualifying as a doctor. Many large hospitals in the US offer specialist fellowship training in joint replacement.

Q **Are special facilities and specialist staff needed for surgery?**

Joint replacement, in particular, requires specialist facilities and the expertise of a hospital. Operating rooms are equipped with ultraclean airflow systems and dedicated orthopedic floors to help maintain hygiene and reduce the risk of infection. Nursing staff are trained to care for the particular needs of people who undergo joint surgery. Physical therapists and occupational therapists are part of the multidisciplinary team working toward effective postoperative recovery and rehabilitation.

JOINT SURGERY

Orthopedic surgeons have a number of treatment options to choose from, depending on the particular problem that affects your arthritic joint. Generally speaking, they all aim to relieve pain or prolong the life of a joint. The main types of joint surgery available include washing out, synovectomy, realignment, fusion, and total joint replacement. The chart below summarizes the purpose of each type.

TYPE OF SURGERY	PURPOSE	EFFECT
Washing out	To remove loose fragments from inside a joint such as the knee	To relieve pain
Synovectomy	To remove the synovium (membrane lining a joint) from an inflamed joint	To slow the overall arthritic process
Realignment	To correct a deformity or straighten a limb	To relieve pain
Fusion	To prevent joint movement	To relieve pain
Joint replacement	To replace all or part of a joint, such as the hip, with an implant	To relieve pain and restore movement
Spinal surgery	To relieve pressure on the spinal cord, to fuse adjacent vertebrae, or to remove an affected intervertebral disk	To relieve pain

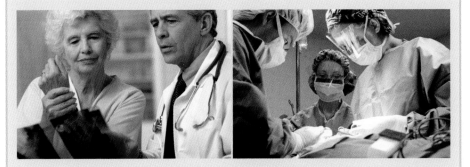

Q I have been offered minimally invasive surgery as a surgical option. What are the benefits and risks?

Minimally invasive surgery (MIS) reduces the size of incisions as a way of limiting blood loss and muscle damage during an operation. It may also speed up recovery from joint replacement. However, there is some doubt about whether MIS for hip or knee replacement is as good as conventional methods. Potential risks of MIS include fractures of the thighbone and nerve injury. Before agreeing to have such surgery, you should find out how long your surgeon has been using MIS and what his or her success rate is.

Q My doctor tells me I have osteoarthritis of my left knee and I need to have it realigned. What does this involve?

Osteoarthritis of the knee mainly affects the inner part of the joint and may be associated with a bowlegged appearance of the legs. As the arthritis progresses, more and more load from the body's weight is transferred down through the inner part of the knee. A surgical realignment of the joint (also called osteotomy, see box p99) can, in some cases, reverse this deformity. The procedure can often relieve pain and delay the progression of arthritis.

Q Various tests and scans have revealed arthritis in my spine—what are the surgical options available to me?

Many types of arthritis can affect the vertebrae of the spine so it depends on what is causing your problem. Surgery cannot eliminate the arthritis itself. However, if bony spurs in osteoarthritis have restricted the space for the spinal cord or a spinal nerve, your surgeon might use a procedure called decompression to widen the space. If the disk between two vertebrae is diseased, the surgeon might remove it and might fuse the vertebrae, but this operation does not guarantee that all your pain will be eliminated.

Q My doctor says I have loose fragments in my knee and the joint needs washing out. What does this involve?

A surgeon introduces an arthroscope (a fiberoptic tube with a microchip camera) through a tiny incision into the joint to look at the bone surfaces, cartilage, and ligaments. Tiny instruments guided by the arthroscope, such as forceps, are used to remove the fragments and roughen the exposed bone on the surfaces of the joint (a process called chondroplasty) in order to stimulate new cartilage formation. Fluid can be injected into the joint and removed, together with loose debris, using a vacuum. This process is sometimes called arthroscopic lavage.

OSTEOTOMY OF THE KNEE

In the realignment, or osteotomy, of a knee, the surgeon cuts through the shinbone (tibia) and wedges bone graft into the incision. A metal plate is attached to the bone with screws to hold the incision open. The procedure straightens the leg so that the force across the knee passes through the middle of the joint instead of the inner part. As a result, the load of the body on the knee is spread evenly across the entire joint. After surgery, regular physical therapy keeps the knee functioning until full range of motion is restored. This rehabilitation process after surgery usually takes between 3 and 6 months.

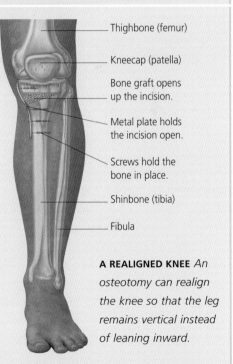

Thighbone (femur)

Kneecap (patella)

Bone graft opens up the incision.

Metal plate holds the incision open.

Screws hold the bone in place.

Shinbone (tibia)

Fibula

A REALIGNED KNEE *An osteotomy can realign the knee so that the leg remains vertical instead of leaning inward.*

Joint replacement

Q **If I have a total joint replacement will I lose some mobility or flexibility in the joint?**

It depends on which joint is being replaced. If the joint being replaced is the hip or knee, there usually is no loss of mobility or flexibility. However, replacing other joints, such as the shoulder, may not be as successful at maintaining mobility and flexibility.

Q **How successful are total hip replacements?**

If you are in constant pain, unable to move, and wholly dependent on others, then a total hip replacement (see p103) can transform you into a pain-free, mobile, and independent person. Over 165,000 total hip replacement operations are performed in the US each year, and over 90 percent are entirely successful. According to the American Academy of Orthopedic Surgery, total hip replacement should have an 80 percent chance or better of lasting 20 years or more in people aged 65 or above. In actual fact, many well-established designs of total hip replacement last much longer than this.

Q **Can I have a hip joint resurfaced rather than replaced?**

Yes, if that's what you and your surgeon agree is best. People with a resurfaced hip often regain a very good range of safe movement. Whether these resurfacing techniques will outlast conventional hip replacements remains to be seen.

Q **I'm an active 35-year-old but I have osteoarthritis in my hip. Am I too young for a replacement?**

No. You may be a good candidate for a total hip replacement because techniques and implants have improved so much that they are as suitable for younger, more active people as they are for older, less active people.

Q I have rheumatoid arthritis in my left shoulder—can it be replaced?

Yes, you can have a half-joint replacement (hemiarthroplasty) of the ball of the shoulder joint. This procedure can produce good results. The rotator cuff muscles, which are very important in stabilizing the joint, are often in poor shape in rheumatoid arthritis so a hemiarthroplasty is usually effective for alleviating pain. The operation may not improve the shoulder's range of movement, but the joint should feel much more comfortable.

Q I have osteoarthritis in my right shoulder—can it be replaced?

Yes, you can have a total shoulder replacement, which is usually performed when the joint is affected by osteoarthritis. The success of this procedure often depends on how much bone is available in the socket, which is usually the component that surgeons find most difficult to fix securely.

Q Osteoarthritis is affecting my left knee. Can I have the whole knee replaced with an implant?

Yes, you can, although it will depend on how your knee is affected and which part is involved. Modern knee designs for total knee replacements (see p104) are very effective in alleviating pain. The risks are very similar to those for total hip replacement, so it is important that you discuss these with your surgeon before deciding to have the operation. Individual parts of the knee can be replaced, too. The most common operation is the unicompartmental replacement of the inner side of the knee. Such implants, which replace only one part, can often last 10 years or more. Less common is the replacement of the patello-femoral joint (the joint between the kneecap and the knee), although it is too early to say how successful this procedure will be in the long term.

Total knee and hip replacements

The total replacement of an arthritic hip or knee are among the most effective treatments and surgical success stories in modern medicine. A combination of surgical expertise and technological innovation have made it possible to replace whole joints with implants made of strong, frictionless materials that the body does not reject but accepts as its own.

TOTAL KNEE REPLACEMENT

In a total knee replacement, the surgeon moves the kneecap to one side to expose the joint surfaces. He or she removes the diseased cartilage and makes precise cuts in the bone to receive the metal caps. These caps are very accurately positioned and attached to the top of the shinbone —either with or without cement—and to the bottom of the thighbone. The caps are shaped like the natural knee to allow free and easy movement. A plastic spacer placed in between keeps friction low and allows free movement without loosening the implant. The kneecap surface may also be replaced with a plastic insert.

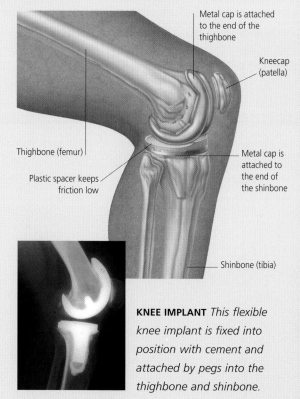

Metal cap is attached to the end of the thighbone

Kneecap (patella)

Thighbone (femur)

Plastic spacer keeps friction low

Metal cap is attached to the end of the shinbone

Shinbone (tibia)

KNEE IMPLANT *This flexible knee implant is fixed into position with cement and attached by pegs into the thighbone and shinbone.*

TOTAL HIP REPLACEMENT

In a total hip replacement operation, the damaged ball-and-socket components of the hip are removed and replaced with artificial implants, which may be secured with or without cement. After removing the diseased ball and the diseased cartilage lining the socket, the surgeon securely and precisely positions an artificial cup with a very smooth inner plastic lining into the socket and ensures that the joint remains stable after the operation. He or she inserts an artificial stem into the thighbone and fits a metal or ceramic ball to the top. The surgeon places the new ball into the prepared socket and carefully reattaches the muscles around the top end of the thighbone.

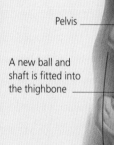

Pelvis

A new ball and shaft is fitted into the thighbone

Skin incision is usually 4–5in (10–25cm) long

The center of the thighbone shaft is hollowed out using a reaming device

A new cup with a smooth plastic lining is fitted in the hip socket

THE ARTIFICIAL JOINT *The new ball may be made of metal, although modern implants increasingly use durable ceramics that are smoother and wear better in the long term.*

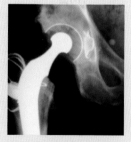

THE IMPLANT IN PLACE *An X-ray reveals a new hip implant in position, with the stem inside the thighbone and the ball sitting in the plastic cup.*

Before and after surgery

Q I've just received a letter confirming the date of my operation. How can I best get fit for surgery and prepare for a stay in the hospital?

First, you should exercise as much as you can to improve your fitness and strengthen the muscles around your joints. If you have breathing problems, such as asthma, try to make sure your chest is in a good condition. If you're a smoker, stop smoking. If you are overweight, try to shed some extra pounds. Try to keep free from infections; this includes dealing with bad or loose teeth and infected toenails. If you are a woman and on oral contraceptives or hormone therapy (HT), you may wish to stop taking it because it increases the risk of a blood clot. Get in touch with your surgeon or doctor to find out more information.

Q Should I consider making arrangements for the time I need to recover from my operation?

Yes. Before you undergo surgery, it is important to think about what life will be like after you have recovered. Discuss with your surgeon the restrictions you may need to impose on your work and lifestyle activities. Find out what benefits you are entitled to, ask an occupational therapist what aids you may need, and talk to your family and friends about organizing help around the home.

Q Will I have to take time off from work?

Almost certainly. Talk to your employer before you plan time off for surgery, so they know well in advance. Discuss your eligibility for sick pay and any modifications you may need when you return (see p118). You will probably be able to return to a sedentary job in 6–8 weeks after joint replacement surgery, but full function may not be achieved for 12 weeks.

Q I've been told I have to attend a preoperative assessment clinic. What tests can I expect to have and what forms do I need to sign?

A preoperative clinic is a vital part of the preparation for your surgery. You will meet your surgeon, who will assess potential risk factors, such as high blood pressure, and take steps to treat such problems before surgery. You will have to sign a consent form. The team will take your detailed medical history, conduct routine blood tests, and may record an electrocardiograph (ECG) to check the condition of your heart. They may also take X-rays of your troublesome joint. A physical therapist and an occupational therapist will discuss your rehabilitation and suggest possible modifications to your home.

Q I've heard that an occupational therapist will advise me on what changes I might need to make to my home. Is this true?

Yes. At the preoperative assessment clinic, the occupational therapist will be particularly concerned that any modifications to your home are done before your discharge. For example, you may need handrails fitted beside your bath or shower or extra banisters installed on the stairs. If you are undergoing a total hip or knee replacement, your seats and chairs, even the toilet seats, at home may need to be raised before you return. The Arthritis Foundation can advise you further on equipment and aids (see Useful addresses, p184).

Q What do I need to take with me to the hospital?

It is important to bring everything you need to make your stay in the hospital as comfortable as possible: dressing gown, nightwear, toiletries, plenty of reading material, and perhaps a personal CD player or radio. Bring several changes of clothing because you will be encouraged to get back into your everyday clothes as soon as possible after your surgery.

Q Will I get a chance to talk to my surgeon and anesthetist?

Yes. Once you are comfortable in the ward, a member of the surgical team will visit you and mark the joint that needs surgery as a fail-safe mechanism to avoid mistakes. Your surgeon will pay you a visit to make sure everything is in order. Your anesthetist will discuss exactly what technique is best for you, depending upon whether you want to be awake or not during the procedure, and taking into account any other medical factors or previous anesthetic problems.

Q I would like to stay awake during my operation so that I can watch—is this a good idea and what sort of anesthetic will I need?

Talk to your surgeon about this, as well as other people who have watched their own operation, before you make up your mind. Watching the operation may make you feel nauseous and increase your anxiety. On the other hand, it may comfort you to feel a part of what is going on. If you do decide to watch, you will be given a local anesthetic so that only the area around the site of the operation becomes numb.

Q What happens on the day of surgery?

Before you are due to go to the operating room, your surgeon will visit you for a preoperative talk. If there is anything more you need to know about the operation, now is the time to ask. When the time comes for your surgery, you will put on a sterilized gown and remove all jewellery (except wedding rings), nail polish, and dentures. You may be given premedication to relax you. You will be taken from the orthopedic floor to the operating room reception either in a wheelchair or on a gurney. You then go to the anesthetic room outside the operating room where you will see your anesthetist again and your surgeon will check you over just before the operation begins.

Q What can I expect when I wake up after the operation?

Once the operation is over, you will be brought back to the recovery room. You will have an intravenous drip in one of your arms, and you may have drain tubes connected to drain bags, which collect any blood lost after the operation. These will be removed within 24 hours. You should wake up after the operation with little or no pain. You will probably return to the orthopedic floor within an hour or two of the operation, and later in the day you should be able to have short visits from friends or relatives.

Q I have just had surgery on my knee—what recovery milestones do I need to reach before I can leave the hospital and go home?

The hospital staff need to make sure that you are safe to go home so you will need to demonstrate that you can walk safely with crutches or a walker, can get into and out of bed, and into and out of a chair. Your physical therapist will check if you can negotiate stairs and steps. He or she will want to see if the muscles around the knee are recovering and to know you have regained a good range of movement prior to your discharge.

Q What checks will be made when I am discharged from the hospital?

Discharge planning is important to make sure the outcome of your operation is as good as possible. Dissolving stitches are often used by surgeons to close incisions, but if you have stitches (sutures or staples) that need removing, plans for their removal—either at your doctor's office or at the rehabilitation facility—will be made. At the time of discharge, checks will be made to ensure that all the necessary modifications to your home are in place, and that any social services care is ready for you when you get home. The hospital should also give you contact numbers to call if you do have any problems after your discharge.

Myth "Knee replacements are not as good as hip replacements"

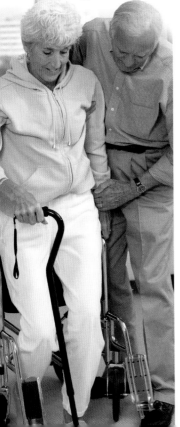

Truth   This used to be the case 15 or 20 years ago when knee replacement designs were very basic. Today, however, the introduction of new designs of implant that more closely simulate the movement and structure of the natural knee have revolutionized the procedure so that knee replacements last just as long as hip replacements, and might be doing even better.

Returning home

What sort of postoperative care will I need?

Everybody who has surgery for arthritis will need some sort of help after the operation, even those who are young and fit, because of the fatigue they will inevitably feel. Discuss this in detail at the preoperative assessment visit so that appropriate arrangements can be made. After joint replacement surgery, elderly people will require much more care from family, friends, and social services. In some circumstances, a short period of convalescence in a suitable nursing home may be necessary after your discharge from the hospital.

I have just returned home after a total knee replacement. What rehabilitation milestones will I need to reach before I can return to work?

You will probably have to keep using your crutches for perhaps 4–6 weeks after the operation in order to avoid excessive load on the implant. This period may seem like a long time but it will give both your muscles and your wound a chance to heal well. You will then start coming off crutches gradually, perhaps on to a cane, but you should notice your level of mobility will improve steadily. As long as you do not have other joint problems, you will probably be able to come off canes and crutches completely by 10–12 weeks after the operation. At this stage you should be walking freely and really starting to get back to a normal life.

After having a total hip replacement, should I be doing some exercises?

During your rehabilitation from a total hip replacement, it is important to try to walk a little each day because this will help your recovery and also minimize the swelling in your leg.

THE LIFESPAN OF REPLACEMENT JOINTS

Replacing joints, or arthroplasty, is the mainstay of surgical treatment for arthritis because artificial joints can provide many years of stable and pain-free movement. Some joints, such as the knee, hip, and shoulder, can also be partially replaced. The success of total joint replacement is due to improvements in surgical techniques, the methods of fixing the implants in position, and the implants themselves. Almost every joint in the body can be replaced, although some replacements are more successful than others and have a longer lifespan.

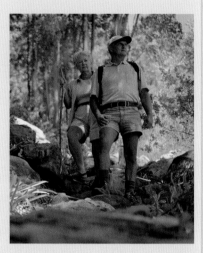

JOINT	TYPE OF ARTHRITIS	PROGNOSIS	LIFESPAN
Hip	All types	Very good	Should last 15 years or more
Shoulder	All types	Good	Should last 10 years
Shoulder (partial)	Rheumatoid arthritis	Good	Should last 10 years
Knee	All types	Very good	Should last 15 years or more
Elbow	Rheumatoid arthritis	Good	Should last 10 years
Knuckle	Rheumatoid arthritis	Good	Should last 5–10 years
Ankle	Rheumatoid arthritis	Unknown	May last 5 or more years

Q After a total replacement of a hip or knee, how long will it be before I can drive?

Discuss with your surgeon when you can return to driving a car, although it is usual to wait for perhaps 4–6 weeks after lower limb joint replacement surgery. You will be able to undertake short trips in a car as a passenger almost immediately after discharge from the hospital, but if you need to make any longer trips within the first 12 weeks after surgery, you should stop regularly to get out and stretch your legs.

Q How soon will I be able to fly after surgery?

It is probably not a good idea to fly until 12 weeks have passed after your surgery because of the slightly increased risks of blood clots (deep vein thrombosis). Many people notice that their joints continue to improve for at least 12 months after the operation, at which stage they may feel that they never had the operation.

Q What kind of complications might occur after surgery?

A few complications can develop after any surgery and during rehabilitation. The risks that are particular to the surgery of arthritis include infection, blood clots, and dislocation (see p112). Nerve injury and excessive bleeding are rare complications, which your surgeon will probably explain to you at the preassessment visit (see p105).

Q What happens if my implant becomes infected?

The risk of infection is not high in total joint replacements —only about 1 in 200 cases. Surgeons make every effort to reduce the risk of infection. You are given antibiotics and the operation is performed in an ultraclean operating room by a team wearing special surgical suits. Nevertheless, infection in an implant or bone can be very difficult to treat. The only way is to remove the infected implant to let the infection clear, then insert a new implant.

Q What are my chances of developing a blood clot?

The risk of a serious blood clot developing in one of your legs is about 1 in 100, especially after an operation on your legs or pelvis. Reducing your weight before surgery, and getting your mobility back soon after surgery, can lower the risk. A blood-thinning agent such as heparin can help prevent blood clots, too.

Q If I take a blood-thinning agent, what happens if I cut myself?

You should contact your doctor at once if you cut yourself, have a nosebleed, or notice blood in your urine. Your doctor will probably prescribe a drug that helps your blood clot.

Q What are the chances of my implant becoming dislocated?

If you've had a total hip replacement, there's a small risk that the new joint may dislocate, and the ball and socket come apart. This risk, probably only 1 or 2 in 100, is highest in the first 6–12 weeks after your operation. If you have had a total hip replacement, don't cross your legs or bend over too far too soon. Follow the advice of your physical therapist and protect your limb from any situation where dislocation may occur. Of course, you can use your new joint for its entire lifetime, but respect it and avoid overloading it repeatedly or forcing it into awkward positions.

Q How long will my replacement be expected to last?

A replacement joint should last for many years, especially if you look after it (see box, p110). Studies of large numbers of people with joint replacements give statistical chances of how long a joint will last. For example, data from Sweden suggests that many hip replacements have a better than 80 percent chance of lasting 20 years or more, before they need to be replaced by revision surgery (see p113).

Q Can an artificial joint eventually work its way loose?

Yes, it can. If you have had a joint replaced, and then it begins to fail, it is usually because the implant loosens inside the bone. The load-bearing surface of the implant also wears out slowly. This is to be expected because a hip or knee may go through a million movements each year in normal use. As a result, you may be a candidate for revision surgery and a new joint. As the joint loosens, it might become painful. Sometimes, a joint can loosen without pain so you are unaware that the bone around your implant is becoming very thin. For this reason, your joint replacement should be X-rayed every 5 years or so, even if you feel fine.

Q Will I need to have the artificial joint replaced in the future?

Possibly. It depends how old you are and how active your life is. The younger you are when your hip or knee is replaced, the shorter time it is likely to last, since younger people use their joints more vigorously. Elderly people who have joints replaced may never need to have them revised. Revision surgery is not to be undertaken lightly—it takes longer and is technically demanding. Nevertheless, a successfully revised joint can perform almost as well as the first one, giving you back your mobility and independence.

Q What are the risks of revision surgery?

The risks are usually higher than those for primary operations. Candidates for revision surgery are older than when they had their first joint replacement operation and their general health may not be as good. For each subsequent revision operation, the risks of infection go up and the amount of blood loss can be greater. The muscles, ligaments, and skin become more scarred and fail to heal as well.

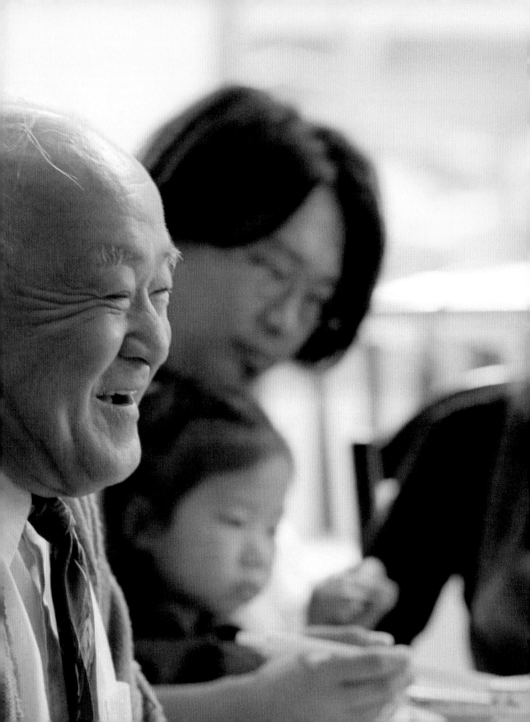

Living with arthritis

People with arthritis need to make changes in their lifestyle. Minor adjustments may be all that's required; but if you are severely affected, you may have to make profound changes. Many specialists can guide and advise you on issues, such as work, domestic activities, driving, family life, and personal relationships. Yet, it is important to be able to manage your own arthritis, to protect your joints, and to know how to cope with flare-ups and stress.

At work

Q How will arthritis affect the way I work?

The pain, stiffness, and other symptoms can have a profound impact on the way you go about your work, but it depends on what kind of arthritis you have and how severe it is. Obviously, it also depends on the type of work you do, particularly if your work involves physical activity of some kind. You probably will be worried about finances, how sympathetic your employer will be, or how you are going to perform. The best thing to do is talk to your employer and try to resolve any issues together.

Q Does having arthritis mean that I have to give up work?

Not usually, although you might have to take time off work if you need treatment such as surgery. You may also find that some days are worse than others and you may occasionally have to call in sick. If arthritis does not compromise your job excessively, it is important to identify and resolve potential problems as early as possible. It is always best to keep your employer informed, and to figure out ways that help you continue at work. If you can't sort things out with your employer, seek independent advice (see p117).

Q Is there any special advice for people with inflammatory arthritis?

Don't make hasty decisions about giving up work. Have a frank discussion with your rheumatologist or rheumatology nurse about whether you are on the most effective medication. Use self-management methods (such as joint protection, fatigue management, exercise, and splints), wait for your medication to become as effective as possible, and make changes to your work. Then you can make realistic decisions about your future.

Q **What help can I get if I did have to stop work altogether—even for a while?**

Occupational therapists, physical therapists, and many other specialists can provide you with a great deal of advice and guidance to help you manage your arthritis and deal with everyday issues. The Disability Employment Agency (DEA) can also advise you on future employment options and about benefits available, to support you financially. You can also get advice about benefits from the Social Security Administration.

Q **What can I do if I have to give up work?**

Stopping work affects people differently. You may feel a loss of self-confidence and self-worth. So, plan your activities for the coming week. Even if it's just for a few hours a week, doing volunteer or community work, studying (online or local adult education classes), or further training, will give you something to look forward to. It also demonstrates to future employers that you have continued to use or develop skills, even though you needed to take a break from work. If you can't do these activities, pursue hobbies to keep your mind active and to ensure meaning and purpose in life.

Q **What legal requirements does my employer have to abide by?**

Under US law, you have certain rights. If, for example, you have rheumatoid arthritis, you should not have to worry about being fired because of your condition. The Americans with Disabilities Act (1990) states that your employer is responsible for making reasonable accommodations to your current job or considering you for suitable vacancies within the company. However, you must educate yourself about your rights uder the Occupational Safety and Health Act (1970) and the ADA Accessibility Guidelines for Buildings and Facilities (1991, amended 2002).

Q **Arthritis makes it hard to do some aspects of my work. How can my workplace be modified to accommodate this?**

Under the law, your place of employment should be accessible to anyone with a disability. Your employer also has a duty to make "reasonable accommodations" that are affordable and will not cause disproportionate disruption to the business. These include changes to your working environment, duties, and timetable, and the purchase of modified equipment and assistive devices. You may even be assigned a support worker to help you get the job done.

Q **I'm concerned my employer won't abide by the requirements of the law. What should I do?**

If you are concerned your employer will not abide by such requirements, seek advice and support—for example, from your union or Disability Employment Agency. Ask to be referred for an occupational health assessment. Most companies and organizations can access doctors or nurses; a few also employ counselors, physical therapists, and occupational therapists. They can also advise on workplace modifications.

Q **I just took several months off sick. How can I make a successful return to work?**

If you have been off work for surgery, or perhaps had to take a few months off because of your rheumatoid arthritis, a successful return can depend on factors like the nature of your job, the severity of your arthritis, and how long you have been away. Tell your employer about your arthritis and discuss the kind of changes needed. Suggest a graded return in terms of a build-up of hours and responsibilities, and ask for a regular review. If you can only manage a few hours, estimate the minimum income you need to decide how much to work per week. Your occupational therapist can support you and the Disability Employment Agency can help you negotiate changes and work-related benefits.

Asking for help

Q **What help can an occupational therapist give me now that I have been diagnosed with arthritis?**

Occupational therapists can help you achieve your personal, professional, domestic, educational, or leisure goals. They can help you improve your ability to carry out routine tasks, make lifestyle changes, and prevent or reduce your chances of losing your abilities in the future. They can advise you on household chores, home modifications, and assistive devices.

Q **Can occupational therapists teach me how to look after my joints?**

Yes. They can show you how arthritis affects your joints, and how you can simplify your day-to-day activities. Occupational therapists can also teach you physical and psychological techniques to manage your pain and fatigue. They can even make splints to rest and support painful or damaged joints.

Q **How can I get in touch with a local occupational therapist?**

A rheumatologist can refer you to a rheumatology occupational therapist who specializes in solving the problems of arthritis. Either on your own or through a referral from your health professional, you can contact an occupational therapist at a local clinic for advice on larger equipment or home adaptations.

Q **I'm afraid to ask for help because it feels as though I'm giving in to arthritis. Does everyone feel this way?**

Many people are reluctant to ask for help yet there is no point in being worried or shy. In fact, make sure you try to get all the help you need to manage your life more effectively. You don't have to fight your arthritis alone. Don't be afraid to ask for help. Acknowledge your changed circumstances and accept help without feeling guilty.

At home

Q **Household chores really make my joints ache and feel sore. What can I do to make things easier?**

Bending, lifting, pushing, gripping, and carrying objects while doing household chores can take their toll on sore and aching joints and leave you with little energy to enjoy leisure activities. Think of easier ways of doing things. Try sitting while preparing food. Use energy-saving equipment, such as a microwave. Well-designed tools require less effort to use and are less stressful for your joints. A good example is the chunky grip on hand tools or on lever door handles and faucets. If you have painful wrists or knees, wear a supportive splint.

Q **I find cleaning causes me pain, especially when I have to bend down. How can I make cleaning less painful?**

Try to keep an upright posture, bend your knees rather than your back, and don't try to clean the whole house in one session. A lightweight, upright vacuum cleaner may be easier to use. Make sure you can grip the handle, operate the controls, and change the bags easily before you buy one. Ask someone to carry the vacuum cleaner upstairs or, better still, keep another one up there permanently. Bending to pick items can be difficult. So a reacher or long-handled dustpan and brush can be useful. To save on trips upstairs when neatening up, collect items in a basket at the bottom of the stairs and take them up in one trip.

Q **Are there easier ways of making beds, especially doing up the comforter covers?**

Stretchable man-made fabrics, fitted sheets, and lightweight comforters may be easier to manage. You can also use velcro fastenings on covers because they are kinder to hands rather than snaps.

Are there tips to help me do the washing and ironing?

Front-loading washing machines and tumble driers are easier to reach if mounted on a firm platform. Use push-on clothes pins rather than squeeze-open ones to clip clothes on a line. If you find reaching up difficult, try propping up your clothes line. The line can be let down to hang on the clothes and then raised up to dry. When ironing, wear a wrist support, use a lightweight iron, and sit on a stool (see p176). Iron a little at a time. Many man-made fabrics do not need to be ironed at all.

COPING WITH HOUSEWORK

Cleaning, neatening, making meals, doing the laundry, ironing, and all those other chores that constitute household work can be tiring at the best of times. There are a number of tips that will conserve your energy, protect your joints, and generally make your life a good deal easier.

TIP	ACTIVITY
Plan ahead	Make a list of household jobs and do a little over several days, rather than all at once. Plan rest days and organize potential helpers.
Pace yourself	Take regular breaks when doing housework. Be systematic and avoid unnecessary trips around the house and upstairs.
Watch your posture	Keep a relaxed upright posture; bend from the knees rather than the back. Change position often and avoid gripping things tightly for long periods—for example, when polishing or scrubbing pans.
Get help	Ask family or friends to help with heavier tasks. You may be able to pay someone to do the cleaning for you.
Keep things handy	Store often-used items at the front of cabinets at chest height. Throw away bottles you don't use. Keep cabinets uncluttered.

Q **Arthritis affects my hands and causes problems when I prepare meals. Are there tips and devices to help me in the kitchen?**

If you cook often, and you can afford to, buy lightweight power tools to stir, chop, grate, and whisk food. Use a knife and vegetable peeler with a chunky grip. Choose appliances, such as an oven and a microwave, that you can reach into and that feature easy-to-operate controls. Use lightweight pans, preferably with two handles, for cooking. To avoid lifting pans of boiling water, steam or microwave your vegetables. If you use a saucepan, put a french fry basket in the pan. When the vegetables are done, you can remove the basket and leave the pan of water to cool. Alternatively, use a slotted spoon. If you do not eat in the kitchen, a cart can be helpful to carry food to another room. Keep some frozen meals at hand for "bad days".

Q **Arthritis makes shopping much harder than it used to be. How can I make it less stressful?**

Internet shopping and home-delivery services have made this job easier for many people. Most supermarkets will pack groceries and take them to your car. Supermarkets also have shallow clip-on carts that are compatible with wheelchairs. Disabled parking places are available near most stores, banks, and offices.

Q **I used to love gardening but now arthritis makes me reluctant to do anything but the most simple tasks. Are there ways I can start again?**

There's no need to forego the pleasures that gardening brings you. You can successfully do most of the gardening activities you used to love, and you can carry out many of the maintenance tasks needed to keep your garden looking beautiful. Adapt the ideas on coping with housework (see box, p121) and use ergonomic or adapted gardening tools whenever and wherever you can (ask for advice at your local garden center). Use a kneeler seat to save bending. Make sure you pace yourself by alternating your gardening with periods of rest, and plan your activities efficiently.

Q **Would wearing a splint help me with my everyday tasks?**

Wearing a splint can support and protect unstable and painful joints in your body, such as the wrists, hands, fingers, knees, and ankles. Splints can help you with walking, gripping, handling objects, and in easing the pain and swelling of arthritis. You can either buy them "off the shelf" or ask an occupational therapist or a physical therapist to design one that meets all of your requirements.

SOLVING EVERYDAY PROBLEMS

Assistive devices are based on common sense or are the result of ingenious solutions. They are derived from tried-and-tested ways of helping you solve manual problems and fulfill everyday activities that are normal for people without arthritis.

ACTIVITY	PROBLEM	SOLUTION
Writing	Weak grip due to painful wrist and fingers	Use a pen with a chunky rubber grip and relax your grip on the pen as you write.
Peeling potatoes	Gripping and turning the peeler	Choose a wide-handled peeler (available in department stores).
Washing and drying feet, neck, and back	Reaching becomes difficult due to pain.	Wash with a long-handled sponge; dry with lightweight towel with hand loops; and wear a terrycloth bathrobe.
Picking up things from the floor	Reaching down	Use a reacher.
Turning a key	Gripping and turning a key	Fit a handle to your key to give yourself better leverage.

Assistive devices

Using assistive devices or gadgets will help you cope with the difficulties that arthritis can cause. These devices may be familiar products that you can find in most drug stores or in stores that specialize in products designed to help overcome a disability. For example, electric can-openers are widely available and reduce the effort required by a manual can-opener. However, you will need to find a specialist store or supplier to purchase a sock aid (which helps put socks on when you cannot reach your feet). The Arthritis Foundation can advise you on equipment and aids.

CHOOSING ASSISTIVE DEVICES

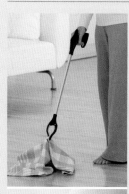

PICK-UP TOOL *You can avoid the pain of bending down to pick things up off the floor if you use a pick-up tool such as a reacher.*

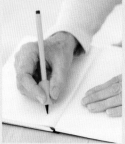

PEN GRIP *Writing is easier with a pen grip because you don't have to press as hard, so you will experience less pain and fatigue.*

Try out an assistive device before buying it. Make sure that mail order products are returnable if found unsuitable. Here are some tips for choosing the right device:

- Pick lightweight, well-crafted products with good grip and easy controls.
- Select devices with chunky handles—they increase leverage and improve grip.
- Consider the posture you'll adopt in order to use the device. For example, a vacuum cleaner with an upright handle is easier on the back than one that requires bending.
- Ask your occupational therapist to help you choose and use a device.
- Ask medical supply stores and pharmacies for their advice in finding and purchasing assistive devices.

PERSONAL CARE

Pain and stiffness in your shoulders, back, and hips can make it hard to reach down to put on shoes and socks, or to reach up to brush your hair or put clothes over your head. Various long-handled gadgets will help with most problems—for example, a long-handled shoe horn, sponge, hair brush, and "helping hand." A stick with a hook at one end and a rubber thimble at the other can help hook pants over your feet or push shirts off your shoulders. It is best to choose clothing with few fastenings if your grip is weak. A button hook can be helpful and tying a loop on a zipper gives a better grip. Choose chunky grips or use an electric toothbrush or razor.

ASSISTIVE DEVICES FOR GENERAL HOUSEHOLD NEEDS

A wide range of gadgets are available to help you with many of your general household needs. These include:

- Jar, bottle, and can-openers.
- Wide-handled peelers, chunky cutlery, and ergonomic knives with upright handles.
- Coffee pot tippers.
- Lever gadgets for taps, door handles, keys, and plugs.
- Long-handled dustpan and brush.
- Self-opening scissors.
- Contour grips to turn both knobs and dials.
- Book rests and pen grips.
- Wrist rests, adapted keyboards, and mouse control for computers.

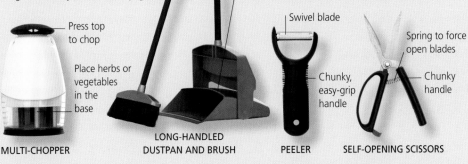

Long handles so you can stand upright

Dust pan swivels so you don't need to bend over

Press top to chop

Place herbs or vegetables in the base

Swivel blade

Spring to force open blades

Chunky, easy-grip handle

Chunky handle

MULTI-CHOPPER

LONG-HANDLED DUSTPAN AND BRUSH

PEELER

SELF-OPENING SCISSORS

Q What modifications can I make to improve the way I get into and around my home?

A grab rail beside the front or back door can help if you have steps. You may need a ramp—a gradient of 1 in 12 is recommended if you use a wheelchair. For the stairs, an extra banister rail may be all you need to steady yourself; for those who need more help, there are many types of stair lifts available on the market and a through-floor elevator will benefit those who use wheelchairs. If you use a walker or wheelchair indoors, you will need a little more space to be able to turn in a room and to move from one room to another. Removing an internal wall can improve your access and mobility in the home. Avoid trips and falls by removing rugs, securing loose carpets, and ensuring that your stairs, hall, and landing are well lit.

Q Arthritis makes it hard for me to sit down and get up from a chair. What can I do to make this easier?

People with arthritis often find that a chair designed with a high seat and back as well as arm-rests is relaxing to sit in. It is also easier to get up from such a chair than from a low couch or sofa. You can raise the seat of your chair by placing a deep cushion on it or by fitting a specially made chair rise unit underneath it. If you are buying a new chair, look for the one with the highest seat that still allows you to place your feet flat on the floor. A powered riser-incliner chair with an elevating leg rest is ideal.

Q Going to the toilet can be awkward and embarrassing. How can I make this more straightforward?

Your toilet needs to be raised, either by building a platform under it or by fitting it with a raised toilet seat, so that you can sit down and stand up more easily. These come with or without rails. A grab rail fitted to the wall may help instead. If arthritis affects your arms and hands, toilets can be equipped with a washing and drying facility. Using moist toilet tissue is easier, too.

Q Is there anything I can do to help me get out of bed more easily?

Beds can be raised up on blocks to help you stand up when you get up. A rail that is fitted to the bed can help you sit up from a lying-down position. Use a supportive, firm mattress. You can obtain even more assistance by using a powered pillow or mattress lifter.

Q How can I adapt my bathroom so that taking a shower or a bath is safe?

Taking a shower is easier than getting in and out of a bath, and a walk-in shower is easiest to access. Either a grab rail on the wall or a seat can be helpful if you do not have a walk-in shower. If you prefer to soak in a warm bath and need more help to get out of the bathtub, try a power-rise bath seat, with or without a reclining back rest.

Q I love cooking but now that I have arthritis, my kitchen seems a difficult place to prepare meals. How can I modify it?

A good ergonomic design in the kitchen may involve altering the height of work surfaces and cabinets, raising or lowering appliances and electric outlets to enable you to gain access easily, and ensuring that controls and handles are easy to grip. The sink, stove, and work surface of your kitchen's "working triangle" should be close together, at the same height, and access to all three should be unobstructed. Keep a stool in the kitchen so that you can rest if you feel tired

Q Who can I turn to for advice about assistive devices and for making modifications to my home?

Look for either a home improvement expert or a local occupational therapist who specializes in home adaptations. Either of them can visit your home and help determine your needs and how these can be resolved. They may also help you fill in any forms—for instance, you may be able to apply for grants to help cover the cost of making your modifications.

Family life and caring for children

Q **Now that I have arthritis, how can I look after my baby safely? How can I change her diapers and give her a bath?**

Pain, fatigue, and disability caused by arthritis can combine to interfere with your role as an active parent. Make sure you can use all the baby equipment safely. Change your baby's diaper somewhere you don't need to stoop. When bathing your baby, use a sculpted foam cushion and nonslip mat. On your "bad" days, just use a mat and a sponge. Try to manage your energy levels so that you have enough to play with your child. Rest as much as you can and conserve energy.

Q **Why do I feel guilty about being unable to do the things I think I should?**

It's not your fault that you can't be active with your children because your knees are so painful, or go out with your partner because you feel too tired. Try not to be so hard on yourself. When the pain and inflammation makes you more irritable, try not to take it out on those nearest to you or push them away when they offer help or comfort.

Q **My family wants to help me but they only seem to make me feel more helpless than I really am. How can I deal with this problem?**

Eager family members can unwittingly contribute to feelings of helplessness, frustration, and dependence. Negotiate the amount of help you want in order to stay as independent as possible. Your family can be a major source of emotional and practical support, so communicate openly with them. They may find it difficult to come to terms with your arthritis, too. Talk about arthritis and how you feel, and encourage questions. This will help them see past the problems to the real you and help them understand the limitations imposed by arthritis.

Arthritis makes me tired and irritable, and I feel as though my relationships are suffering. How can I resolve this?

Arthritis doesn't affect you in isolation—it can potentially affect everyone who comes in contact with you. Good communication is the key to maintaining all relationships—platonic or sexual. Be honest about your feelings with your loved ones. If you can't explain your problems because of arthritis, give them a brochure from the Arthritis Foundation (see Useful addresses, p184).

IMPROVING SEXUAL RELATIONSHIPS

People with arthritis experience the joy and pleasure of loving relationships just like anyone else, but the condition can have a negative impact on sexual relationships because of pain, fatigue, and disability. It is important you address any issues that arise.

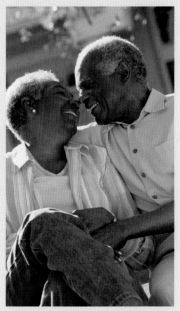

- Paying attention to your whole being is important when you wish to attract others.
- Make time for yourself and your lover, and pamper yourselves.
- Take your medication before sexual activity to be as pain-free as possible.
- Take a hot shower or bath before sexual activity to relax joints and muscles.
- Consider the most convenient method of contraception for you and your partner.
- Find ways to please each other when actual intercourse isn't possible.
- Ask a health professional or a sexual counselor you trust if you cannot resolve your problems.
- Talk to your partner—communication is important for your relationship.

Traveling and moving around

Q The pain and fatigue of arthritis is restricting my independence. Is there anything I can do about it?

When arthritis starts to reduce the frequency and length of time you spend traveling, buy comfortable footwear (such as cross-trainers or thick-soled shoes) and a suitable walking aid (a physical therapist can advise you) to improve your ability to get around. Think about buying a wheelchair or a car with special adaptations.

Q I don't really want to use a scooter or wheelchair—aren't they a sign that I'm just giving in to arthritis?

No, because they can provide you with valuable independence and increase your opportunities to travel and socialize. Standard manual or electric wheelchairs can be covered by Medicaid, Medicare, and standard medical insurance plans if they are medically necessary or the expense may be tax-deductible (ask your doctor to write a prescription). You may also be able to get financial assistance locally, including your employer's charitable program, state vocational rehabilitation offices, and the Department of Veterans Affairs. Try a variety of models before making your choice, and discuss your needs with your occupational and physical therapists.

Q I'm worried that I might have to give up driving my car and lose my independence. What steps can I take to make sure I drive safely?

Driving can be a challenge, depending on the type of car, distance to travel, and severity of your condition. Ask your doctor for the nearest rehabilitation center, where your ability to drive safely will be evaluated. These centers can also recommend special devices that might facilitate your driving, and offer training in using these devices. The Arthritis Foundation produces a helpful brochure, "Driving when you have Arthritis," available on their web site (see p184).

Q How can I make car journeys easier?

Traveling by car can be difficult, but some tips can make the trip easier. For instance, it may help to take your painkillers and/or anti-inflammatory drugs at a particular time before you start so that they are effective when you most need them. Try a wrist support while driving if you have problems with your wrist or grip. Take plenty of breaks during the trip.

Q I need to get a new car soon—is there any help and advice on what is a good type of car to buy?

The car must suit your needs. Make sure it has power-assisted steering, electric windows and mirrors, central locking, and automatic gears. Check that the seat is ergonomically designed and comfortable with adjustable height. Can you get in and out without difficulty? Can you open and close the doors easily and grip the steering wheel firmly? Can you easily operate the hand controls, turn the ignition, and engage and disengage the seatbelt? Once you're sure about all these things, take the car for a couple of test drives before you make up your mind.

Q I have difficulty parking my car near the stores—what assistance can I get?

Under the ADA Accessibility Guidelines for Buildings and Facilities, parking lots must have some parking spaces that are close to the entrance. To use one of these spaces, you must obtain a Disabled Parking placard and display it in your car.

Q Would traveling by bus, plane, boat, or train be better than driving?

These forms of transport can be more relaxing and less stressful than driving a car, especially on long trips. Train stations, ferry terminals, and airports should be accessible under the Americans with Disabilities Act (1990) for people with a disability. It is always worthwhile calling your travel agent to tell him or her what assistance you are likely to need.

Protecting your joints

Q **Why do I need to protect my joints?**

How you stand and move your body affects the stress and strain you place upon your joints. For example, a slouched posture increases the stress on your back and neck. You will put strain on your muscles and joints if you repeat the same movement over and over, or if you hold a joint in the same restricted position for too long. Even using too much effort to do a job can be stressful and tiring. Straining already swollen and painful joints can further weaken their support structures (the ligaments and joint capsules). In time, deformities may develop.

Q **I find it hard to change the habits of a lifetime—do I really need to do things differently?**

Yes, because arthritis can cause some joints to deform over time, creating problems. If you have rheumatoid arthritis, your wrists can start to move downward and your fingers point away from the thumb. In thumb osteoarthritis, a zigzag shape can develop. Many activities, such as lifting, can put a downward pressure or pull on the wrist. Others, such as opening a jar or turning faucets, require twisting movements at the knuckles. Over time, if you have swollen joints, this weakens ligaments and joints start to move in the direction of the pressure. Changing habits is tricky because it takes a great deal of mental effort. Once you get used to analyzing your activities, the ideas will start to multiply.

Q **I'm used to the pain now. Do I need to change my habits?**

People with arthritis often get accustomed to pain, and medication can mask it, so you may not notice an activity causes strain, pain, or fatigue until afterward. So the rule is: if an activity hurts, change it.

KEY PRINCIPLES TO PROTECT YOUR JOINTS

Biomechanics involves the use of efficient physical techniques for standing, moving, and handling objects. Ergonomics is the coordination of tasks and equipment with a person's capabilities. The following key principles use biomechanics and ergonomics to help you protect your joints and manage fatigue.

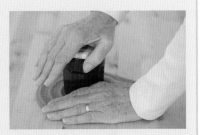

PRINCIPLE	EXAMPLES
Use larger, stronger muscles and joints	If you have hand problems, carry bags over your forearm or shoulder (or use a backpack).
Avoid twisting actions	To open the lid of a jar, press down on it with the palm of the hand (see above) or hold the side of the jar lid between the curve of your thumb and fingers.
Spread the load over several joints	Hold crockery and pots in both palms, rather than with fingers and thumbs.
Use the least effort	Don't grip objects too tightly. Use wheels to move objects. Use assistive devices and labor-saving equipment.
Avoid staying in the same position for too long	If you're sitting for a while, get up and move around for a minute or two every half-hour, or stretch your legs out and move your ankles every few minutes. Take regular breaks from your activities.
Plan your activities more efficiently	Keep everything you need within easy reach and well-organized in drawer dividers, cabinet shelves, and pull-out shelves.
Pace your activities	Do 20 minutes of gardening, for example, then rest for 5–10 minutes.

Q **What does pacing my activities really mean?**

Think of yourself as a battery with a fixed amount of energy for the day. Spend it wisely on what you both need and want to do. Balance periods of rest and activity and give yourself time for leisure and social activities. Regular rests and breaks act as battery rechargers, and regular changes in activity will ease muscle tension. Take a regular break for a few minutes every 30–45 minutes, or at least take a break for 15 minutes every 2 hours. During these breaks, sit down and let your neck and shoulder muscles relax, and let the tension ease away. Physical activity is certainly good for controlling arthritic pain, but so are rest and relaxation.

Q **My doctor said I should rest at regular intervals— but I can't do this at work and I have a family to look after. How can I rest?**

If you can't take a rest break in the day, try microbreaks for 30 seconds every 5 minutes or so, or for 1 or 2 minutes after every 10 minutes. During the break, just briefly stretch the joints and muscles you frequently use, then relax. You could do this at work as well as at home. Train yourself by setting an alarm on a small kitchen timer, your computer, or mobile phone (set it on vibrator mode so it won't annoy others). After a few days, you will find the habit of taking microbreaks starts to form. By taking microbreaks, you won't tire as quickly and can carry on your activity for a longer period of time.

Q **Arthritis is affecting my posture. What is the proper way to stand?**

When you stand, keep your ears in line with your shoulders, which should be relaxed and in line with your hips. Keep your hips in line with your knees and ankles, with your knees very slightly relaxed (not locked rigid), and your weight evenly distributed over your feet.

Q I like to walk a lot—are there things I can do to protect my joints?

First, you need to invest in a good pair of shoes for walking. They should have shock-absorbing soles or insoles, a continuous sole with a slightly beveled heel, and firm support over the top of the foot (laces or straps). Many people with foot and leg problems habitually look down at the ground in front of their feet when walking because they are worried about tripping. Train yourself to look ahead a few yards to help with your posture.

LIFTING A MODERATELY HEAVY OBJECT

Avoid moving and lifting heavy objects whenever possible, particularly if you have knee and hip problems. The steps below will help you safely lift a moderately heavy object. If lifting objects is a part of your job, your employer must, by law, provide you with training and equipment to make this easier.

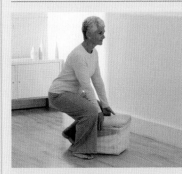

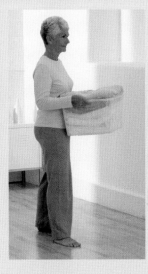

LIFTING THE OBJECT *Make sure that you have a firm hold on the object. Tighten your stomach muscles. Keep the weight close to your body and push upward using your thigh muscles rather than your back muscles.*

GETTING INTO POSITION *To lift a moderately heavy object, first get close to it. Then squat down on your haunches and bend your knees rather than your back.*

Coping with pain

Q What causes pain?

Acute pain is the response of the nervous system when an injury or disease damages the tissues of the body. It's like a simple alarm system that stimulates the body to take protective action to avoid additional damage. However, as anyone who regularly feels pain will tell you, there are types of persistent (chronic) pain that defy all reason and seem to serve no purpose whatsoever.

Q Do we all feel pain the same way?

No. Some people have a low threshold and feel low levels of pain more acutely than others, who seem able to withstand intense pain. It also depends on what is causing the pain and the state of mind you are in—stress, fear, and anxiety can make pain feel worse.

Q How does my body normally cope with pain?

Your body has its own way to relieve pain, at least for short periods. The brain and spinal cord produce endorphins and encephalins, chemicals from the same chemical family as morphine, with a similar sedative effect.

Q Can I learn ways to manage the pain when arthritis flares up instead of relying on drugs?

Yes, it's a good idea to discover ways of coping with your own unique pain. When you get a flare-up, rest —but not in bed. Avoid or reduce activities that aggravate your pain for a couple of days until the pain subsides. Use heat or cold—or whatever you find eases your pain—several times each day. If you feel anxious and tense, practice deep breathing and relaxation exercises. Resume exercising gradually, once the pain starts to settle. If you don't move, your joints will stiffen and your muscles will weaken and tire quickly.

Q **What's the best way to massage a painful joint?**

Massaging and rubbing a painful body part relieves muscle tension, improves circulation, and disperses the fluid in swollen joints and muscles. Gently massaging painful joints or muscles for 5–10 minutes is a very effective, safe, and pleasurable way to relieve pain. Some of the pain relief from moisturizers, lotions, oils, gels, and creams is probably due to the massage that is needed in order to apply them.

Q **Is it true that water therapy can bring pain relief?**

For thousands of years, people have used water therapy to treat arthritic conditions. Water therapy relieves pain by using the warmth and buoyancy of water to relax your muscles and reduce the weight-bearing load and stress on your legs and trunk.

Q **Is spa therapy worth trying?**

This residential treatment involves bathing in naturally heated water, which is often rich in minerals, and applying hot mud packs. Physical treatment is combined with the psychological benefits of receiving respite and care. The effectiveness of spa therapy lies, at least in part, in the absence of domestic pressures, the relaxing environment, and a holistic health approach. However, it is expensive and has limited availability.

Q **What about hydrotherapy or aquatherapy?**

Hydrotherapy is a form of spa therapy that uses the buoyancy, assistance, and resistance properties of warm water to help you exercise effectively. It is a very popular treatment and requires dedicated therapists and specialized facilities. Aquatherapy involves controlled water-based exercises at a moderate cost. You could even exercise gently in your local swimming pool to keep your stiff and painful joints moving.

RELIEVING PAIN WITH HEAT OR COLD

People with arthritis often find that the application of heat or cold can help control the pain of a flare-up. Applying heat is a particularly good way to relax tense and aching muscles. Both heat and cold can improve your blood supply, reduce swelling, and enable you to move around more freely.

HEAT Warmth can be created by commercially available heat packs, a hot-water bottle wrapped in a towel, a hot bath, or thermal clothing or bandages. The resulting warmth can reduce your pain considerably.

COLD Cooling can be produced with commercially available cool packs and coolant sprays. Even a bag of frozen peas wrapped in a towel (see right) can relieve pain, improve the supply of blood, and reduce swelling.

PRECAUTIONS For most people, warming or cooling a joint is a safe technique. However, people who have circulatory problems should consult their doctor, physical therapist, or nurse. Avoid placing wet or frozen items directly against the skin (use a towel wrapped around the item) and make sure you don't burn your skin with a heat pack or hot-water bottle. Whatever method you use, avoid becoming uncomfortably hot or cold.

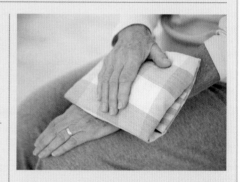

APPLYING HEAT OR COLD Sit or lie down in a comfortable position and relax before applying either heat or cold to the joint. Place the source of heat against the painful, inflamed joint for 10–15 minutes. Remove the source and gently move your joint. The combination of movement and rest is very important for pain relief. Replace the heat pack on the joint for another 5–10 minutes.

To apply cold, place a cool source against the painful, inflamed joint for 10–15 minutes (see above). After removing the pack, move your joint gently to aid the pain relief.

Q **Is it worth buying a TENS machine to help control my pain when it flares up?**

Yes, perhaps, but only after you consult your doctor and learn how to use it from a physical therapist. A TENS (transcutaneous electrical neuromuscular stimulation) machine is a safe, noninvasive way of relieving pain, relaxing tense muscles, and slowing breathing. The device delivers small electrical pulses, via electrodes placed on the skin, that are thought to interfere with pain signals sent to the brain. You can use one at home for about an hour or so, whether you are sitting, standing, or gently moving around. Don't use one if you're pregnant or if you have a pacemaker or heart condition. Never place the electrodes of a TENS machine near the carotid artery in your neck.

Q **Can deep breathing and muscle relaxation exercises provide me with some pain relief?**

Yes, because they help you begin to regain control when the pain seems to be taking over. When you are in pain, you start to think the worst of everything. You become stressed, exacerbate your negative thoughts, and increase your feeling of being helplessly controlled by pain. This vicious circle needs to be broken. At first, you may be sceptical that such simple techniques will help you control pain, but do try them and see. If they don't work, you will have lost little. If they do work, you will gain a great deal.

Q **Could I prevent the pain from developing if I alternated my activities with periods of rest?**

You might. Physical activity is unquestionably good for controlling arthritic pain, as are rest and relaxation. Try to avoid getting tired because it leads to muscle weakness, which increases the risk of further pain and injury. Most people begin to experience pain after doing an activity for a relatively short time, but often continue with the task until it is completed or the pain becomes so bad they are forced to rest. A better solution is to limit the time you spend doing the activity by interspersing it with periods of rest.

Coping with stress

Q I always thought stress was a part of life. Why is it more of a problem for me now?

Sources of stress can be found in changes to your lifestyle, imagined changes (such as fears about the future), and everyday hassles. The effects and symptoms of arthritis are also a source of stress. Stress itself also increases the symptoms of arthritis and contributes to some of your pain, fatigue, muscle tension, and sleep problems.

Q What happens when the stresses in my life accumulate and start to wear me down?

Living with the ups and downs of arthritis can disturb your emotional state so that you may feel frustration, anger, guilt, sadness, loss, fear, anxiety, or hurt. Emotional changes can increase your levels of stress, while your negative thoughts can fuel the vicious cycle of pain, fatigue, and stress. If you believe you can, your response to stress is less likely to be activated. If you believe you can't, or are faced with too many worries and physical problems, you are more likely to be stressed and emotionally upset.

Q How can I change my responses to stress?

You need to release stress before it starts to dominate your life. Many methods can help, including exercise, movement therapies, relaxation, breathing, and meditation. The mind is a powerful tool, too. One advantage of using psychological approaches to stress is that you can control what happens inside your own mind. You can choose how you wish to react to any situation. Our attitudes, thoughts, and beliefs shape our responses to stress, not events, past or present. Changing the way you think takes work and mental effort, especially if you have been under stress for a long time. However, with perseverance, the rewards are a happier outlook in life and better health.

Q How can I identify the negative ways I deal with stress?

The first step toward changing the nature of your stress response is to identify the beliefs and thoughts in your mind. As you become progressively stressed, you get more emotionally upset and are likely to develop automatic negative thoughts (ANTs). These are like thinking traps that pop into your mind involuntarily and, at the time, are very believable. These might include seeing everything in extremes; thinking you know what others are thinking; blaming yourself for events that are not your responsibility; attaching a negative label to an event; pushing aside positive personal experiences and qualities; always thinking you "must" do this and you "should" do that.

Q I don't feel like going out with friends and family any more. The arthritis really gets me down and I'm so tired. If that's how I feel—does it matter?

Yes, it does. But don't blame yourself for feeling this way. It is a common negative thought pattern for people with arthritis. There are positive ways to work through it. Try to figure out a way to break the vicious cycle—develop a logical, rational approach to dispute your negative thoughts and avoid the consequences at the time of the stressful event—to keep yourself from sliding into emotional distress. Such an approach (see pp142–143) will help train your mind toward a more positive, resilient, and effective outlook, so that you are better able to cope with stress-triggering events in the future.

Q What other ways are there to prevent stress from becoming a problem?

Keep a diary to record your exercises, activities, sleep patterns, and the way you solve practical problems. Meditation, deep breathing, and visualization are usually effective for relieving stress, by restoring a more balanced outlook toward life, reducing tension, and lowering blood pressure. Practice them regularly—a daily routine would be ideal.

The ABCDE method

Cognitive therapists and life coaches, who can help us unravel and understand the mental knots and confused thinking that affect us all, have developed very effective strategies for coping with stress. One of these is known at the ABCDE method. The letters ABC are used to help you understand how you respond to a stressful event: A stands for the Activating event, B for the Beliefs and thoughts triggered in your mind, and C summarizes the Consequences (the emotional, physical, or behavioral changes). The letters D for Disputing thoughts and E for Effective actions help you develop strategies to change your response.

THOUGHT-AND-SYMPTOM DIARY

If you commonly experience feelings of stress, keep a thought-and-symptom diary that records the dates of "activating events" that trigger the stress and your responses. Fill it in as soon as you can while the event is fresh in your mind.

Record your thoughts, emotions, and consequences in 3 columns under the headings (A) Activating Event, (B) Beliefs/ Thoughts, and (C) Consequences. This will help you identify the links between your feelings, stress, and arthritic symptoms.

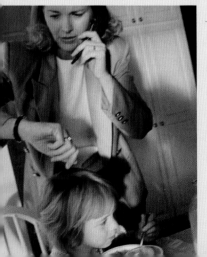

ACTIVATING EVENT

In this example, a woman with rheumatoid arthritis feels stress because her two children won't put on their coats for school and consequently end up rushing to catch the bus.

BELIEFS/THOUGHTS

"I'll never get them to the school bus on time."

"I'm such a terrible mother."

"I can never cope with these kids—I'm useless."

"Every morning is one long struggle."

DEVELOP AN EFFECTIVE OUTLOOK

Once you identify your negative thoughts, try to develop a consciously logical, rational approach to disputing them. Consider the following hints and tips:

- Examine the evidence for your thoughts. Are you applying a double standard to yourself?
- Think in shades of gray, not in all-or-nothing terms. Give different aspects of an event a score on a scale of 0–100.
- Avoid calling yourself names for failing at something. Change the musts and shoulds to cans, and ease up on yourself.
- List the pros and cons of your negative thought, feeling, or behavior. This will help you develop a rational perspective.

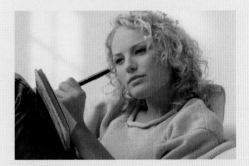

Then, as a positive step to help you change this stress response, create 2 further columns. In the first, record your disputing thoughts that put a positive spin on the event, and in the second, list further actions to take next time.

CONSEQUENCES	DISPUTING THOUGHTS	EFFECTIVE ACTIONS
Feel frustrated, hassled. Tense muscles. Tired.	"Most of the time we manage to get to the bus on time."	Take deep breaths.
Shallow breathing, heart racing, feel stressed.	"Being a little bit late now and then is OK."	Give them a kiss—the kids will want to get away then.
Later in day, pain and fatigue worsen. Worrying.	"I can cope with the kids. Most of the time I do cope perfectly well."	Get lunch ready the night before to avoid having to rush in the morning.
Difficulty in managing so many jobs.		Talk to the kids about why I need them to help.

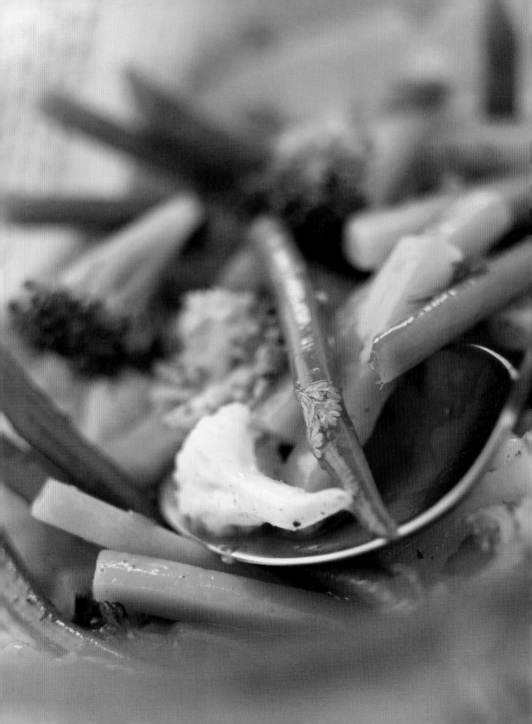

Food and drink

There is a lack of definite medical
evidence to prove that diet can
either trigger the onset of arthritis
or relieve its symptoms. Your doctor
may discourage you from exploring
links between food and your
arthritis for these reasons, but there
are other very good reasons for
paying attention to your everyday
diet. As our understanding of
arthritis progresses, it is becoming
clear that what you eat may have
potential benefits.

Eating a healthy diet

Q Do I have to follow a special diet now that I have been diagnosed with arthritis?

People with arthritis need to eat the type of well-balanced diet that would be a healthy choice for anyone, regardless of his or her age or fitness levels. The most essential components of food are: carbohydrates, protein, fats, vitamins, and minerals. You need some of these essential components in larger quantities than others; the key to a healthy diet is getting the right balance. As a general guide, you should base your diet on fish (white and oily types), poultry, lean red meat, low-fat dairy products, wholegrain or high-fiber cereal foods, lots of fresh fruit and vegetables, including beans and legumes, and only occasionally have greasy, deep-fried, or sugary foods.

Q Should I eat high-fiber, starchy foods and cut down on sugar as part of a healthy diet?

Yes, because carbohydrates are your main source of energy. They are found in starchy foods—such as bread, cereals, rice, pasta, and potatoes—and in sugar. Starchy foods also contain fiber and some nutrients essential to good health, including calcium, iron, and B vitamins. Sugar provides only calories and is of little nutritional value. Starchy foods should make up around a half of what you eat at each meal. Wholegrain or wholemeal varieties of cereals, bread, rice, and pasta are good choices because they contain more fiber than the white varieties. All types of beans and legumes are good sources of fiber, too. Eating high-fiber foods helps keep you feeling fuller for longer and can also help keep your bowels functioning effectively. Try to include some starchy foods in every meal.

How much protein do I need?

Protein helps keep your muscles and other tissues in your body strong and in good working order. Most people need only 2 portions of protein-rich food a day, as well as the milk in cereal, tea, and coffee. Protein foods include dairy products, eggs, beans, legumes, nuts, fish, poultry, and meat. Choose lower fat dairy products and lean meat as an excellent way of avoiding excess calories and fat.

I have a poor appetite and a low body weight. Do I need to eat smaller, protein-rich meals more frequently?

A flare-up of arthritis, especially rheumatoid arthritis, can cause muscle weakness and weight loss, and you may lose your appetite and feel unwell. Eating smaller meals with protein-rich foods more frequently and having protein-rich snacks such as cheese and crackers or milk between meals will help you get the amount of protein you need.

Should I eat unsaturated fat rather than saturated fat?

Generally speaking, yes. Fats come in different forms and some are more beneficial to your health than others, so it is important to know what kind of fat you're eating. The type known as saturated fat is found in fatty red meats and many processed foods—for example, sausages, hard cheese, butter, cakes, cream, coconut oil, and palm oil. As a rule, saturated fat is regarded as an "unhealthy" fat because eating large amounts can increase the level of cholesterol in your blood and contribute to a higher risk of developing heart disease. On the other hand, unsaturated fats found in vegetable oils, particularly safflower, canola, and olive oils, some margarines, and oily fish, are better for you and your heart and for people with arthritis. With so much choice today, it is not difficult or too expensive to eat fats that may be more beneficial to your health. Remember: excess fat of any kind can lead to weight gain.

Q How much fat should I eat?

Fat has more than double the amount of calories we get from carbohydrate or protein. Eating too much fat can lead to weight gain and can increase your risk of developing heart disease. Most packaged foods give the amount of fat in the food on the label. As a general rule, try to choose more foods that contain only a little fat (3g fat or less per 100g) and cut down on foods that contain a lot of fat (20g fat or more per 100g). If the label includes saturated fat, foods with between 1g and 5g contain a moderate amount of saturated fat.

Q Labels on supermarket foods often give the amount of fat as MUFA and PUFA. What is the difference between them?

Both MUFA and PUFA are types of unsaturated fat, so they are considered "healthy." Foods that are rich in MUFAs (monounsaturated fatty acids) include avocados, olive oil, nuts, and seeds, and are thought to help protect against heart disease. There are 2 main groups of PUFAs (polyunsaturated fatty acids) in the diet, called omega-6 and omega-3. You need both, but it is important to get the balance right. Try to increase the amount of omega-3 fats in your diet and eat less omega-6 fats. An easy way to reduce omega-6 fat in your diet is to use olive and canola oils and olive oil-based margarines more often than sunflower-based oils and margarines. Oily fish such as sardines, mackerel, and salmon are an excellent source of omega-3 fats.

Q Would eating a fat-free diet be beneficial?

No, definitely not. All fats and oils provide energy and they are essential to the body's absorption of certain vitamins. The important thing is to eat more foods that are rich in unsaturated fats. These include canola and olive oils, oily fish, avocados, and some nuts (such as almonds and pecan).

Q Will I get any benefits from reducing my intake of salt?

Eating a lot of salt can increase your chance of developing medical conditions such as high blood pressure, heart disease, and stroke. Adults and children over the age of 11 should have no more than 6g (about a teaspoon) of salt a day. Most processed and convenience foods contain large amounts of salt, so eat as much fresh food as you can or choose packaged foods that are low in salt. Low in salt is 0.25g salt or less per 100g. If given as *sodium*, then 0.1g of sodium or less per 100g is considered low. Use just a pinch of salt in cooking and taste your food before adding more salt at the table—you probably won't need it.

Q How much fluid should I drink every day?

More than half of your body weight is made up of water, so drink plenty of fluids. Around 6 to 8 glasses (about 1.5 liters) of fluid a day is sufficient for most people, but this can vary depending on your size and how active you are. Drink plain water if you can, although flavored water (preferably sugar-free), fruit juice, and moderate amounts of tea and coffee count, too. Water or other fluid does not lubricate the joints. However, too little fluid can lead to dehydration, which makes you feel generally unwell and, if you have gout, could trigger an attack.

Q Will drinking alcohol make my symptoms worse?

Not necessarily. There is nothing wrong with having the occasional alcoholic drink, but alcohol is high in calories and regular drinking can contribute to weight gain. If you do drink alcohol, try to keep to the recommended number of units per week—21 units a week for men and 14 units a week for women. Some people with rheumatoid arthritis find that alcohol can provoke symptoms but this is highly individual. However, if you have gout, it is best to avoid alcohol.

Myth "Some foods cause a flare-up in rheumatoid arthritis"

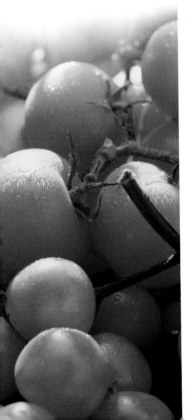

Truth Not necessarily. Several studies show that while food-related flare-ups can occur, only a small percentage of people are affected, and so such reactions are most likely to be coincidental. Common culprits are said to be foods from the nightshade family (potato, tomato, and eggplant) and various peppers and pepper-derived spices (paprika or cayenne). Although a wide variety of foods have been implicated, most people with arthritis do not need to avoid specific foods.

Nutrients to ease arthritis

Q I find the information about nutrients so confusing—which nutrients might help ease the symptoms of arthritis?

There's little solid evidence that individual nutrients can help relieve the symptoms of arthritis, except for omega-3 fats in rheumatoid arthritis. However, eating a varied diet ensures sufficient nutrients to keep you healthy. Eat foods from all food groups: dairy products for calcium and protein; different colored fruit and vegetables for antioxidants and vitamins; fish, lean meat, beans, and legumes for protein; starchy foods for energy and B vitamins; and some MUFA or PUFA for fat-soluble vitamins and energy (see p148).

Q What foods make up the "Mediterranean diet" and would they be good for arthritis?

The Mediterranean diet contains mainly fish and white meats, lots of fresh vegetables and fruit, beans and legumes, olive oil, less dairy products, and a moderate alcohol consumption. Cakes and sweets are not eaten regularly. People with arthritis could benefit from the omega-3 fats from oily fish, less saturated fat, more "good" unsaturated fats from olive oil, and lots of antioxidant vitamins from fresh vegetables and fruits.

Q Will omega-3 fats really help to relieve my pain and inflammation?

Scientific evidence strongly suggests that some "long-chain" omega-3 fats (EPA and DPA) can reduce the pain and inflammation of rheumatoid arthritis. You would need to eat at least 6–7 portions of oily fish a week to get the "useful" amount, which supplements more easily provide (see pp153). Other sources of omega-3 are plant oils, linseeds, and walnuts, but these contain the less effective "short-chain" omega-3 fats.

Helpful supplements

People with arthritis are faced with a huge range of products that may or may not help their symptoms. Some supplements may only help certain kinds of arthritis. The choice of products, coupled with often conflicting stories in the press about their safety and their effectiveness, can make choosing a supplement daunting. Some evidence suggests supplements of glucosamine, chondroitin, fish oils, flaxseed oil, and S-adenosyl-L-methionine may help ease some symptoms of arthritis.

Before you take a product, ask your doctor about its side effects and potentially harmful interactions with other drugs. Only buy brands from reputable companies. Don't mix supplements—find out which ones help and which ones don't. Always take the recommended dosage. Ask your doctor before taking a supplement if you're breast-feeding or pregnant, taking prescription medications, or thinking of giving a supplement to a child.

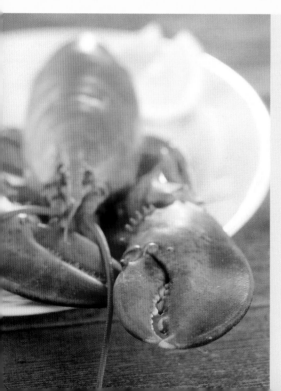

GLUCOSAMINE

An amino sugar found naturally in the body's cartilage, glucosamine may help with joint repair. Several studies have shown that it may ease the pain and stiffness of osteoarthritis, particularly of the knee. If taken for at least 2 weeks, it may be as effective as ibuprofen for pain relief for some people. Glucosamine supplements may be synthetic or include shellfish extracts. The recommended dosage is 750mg, twice a day. Combined with chondroitin it may help some people with moderate to severe knee pain due to osteoarthritis. Avoid glucosamine if you are allergic to shellfish. If you have diabetes, discuss its use with your doctor first.

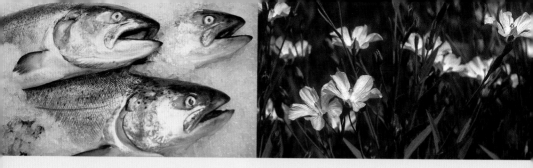

FISH OILS

Fish oil supplements with omega-3 fats in high concentration can relieve some symptoms of rheumatoid arthritis. However, the useful dose is as much as 3g a day. This can be safely achieved with fish *body* oils. Do not take high doses of cod/halibut *liver* oil, which contain vitamin A (retinol), particularly if you are pregnant. High doses of fish oils may cause side effects such as nausea and nosebleeds. Do not take them with anticoagulants such as warfarin.

SAM-e

S-adenosyl-L-methionine (SAM-e) is a natural substance in the body's cells, where it is involved in many metabolic reactions. Although several trials have suggested that SAM-e supplements might have anti-inflammatory and pain-relieving properties, these benefits have not yet been proven in rigorous scientific studies. Avoid high doses, and avoid if you are on antidepressants or MAOIs, or if you have heart disease.

FLAXSEED OIL

Flaxseeds contain an omega-3 fatty acid called alpha linolenic acid (ALA) that the body may convert into the fatty acid EPA, which has anti-inflammatory properties. People can try flax oil as an alternative to fish oils, in capsule form or by adding it directly to food. It is a natural laxative. However, it may interfere with blood-thinning drugs, such as warfarin, and should be avoided by women with uterine cancer or breast cancer.

CHONDROITIN

Chondroitin is found naturally in the body. It is said to lubricate, build, and protect cartilage, and make it more elastic. Studies are ongoing to investigate these claims. The recommended dosage is 600mg, twice a day. If there are no benefits in 3 months, it probably doesn't work for you. If you take warfarin or have a disorder that affects blood clotting, check with your healthcare provider before taking chondroitin.

Q Can plant oils help relieve some of the symptoms of rheumatoid arthritis?

The role that plant oils, such as olive oil, play in fighting arthritis has aroused a great deal of interest. A study has shown that people who consume more olive oil are less likely to develop rheumatoid arthritis. However, there is no evidence that taking lots of olive oil can ease the symptoms of rheumatoid arthritis to the same extent that fish oils can.

Q I've read that taking fish oil is good for rheumatoid arthritis. Does it help osteoarthritis, too?

Evidence suggests that omega-3 fats from fish oils can help relieve the symptoms of rheumatoid arthritis, but there is no conclusive scientific evidence to prove that it also helps ease the symptoms of osteoarthritis. Research into this is still ongoing.

Q I have rheumatoid arthritis. Should I take cod liver oil to help my symptoms and how much do I need to take?

Cod liver oil may help your symptoms but in capsule form it contains far less (long-chain) omega-3 fatty acids than fish body oils. Cod liver oils, in liquid or capsule form, usually contain high concentrations of vitamins A and D. Both of these vitamins are good for you but too much may be harmful. If you take cod liver oil, limit the dose to one capsule a day (of varying size) or two teaspoons (10ml) of oil. Do not exceed the manufacturer's recommendations and avoid taking other supplements that contain high amounts of vitamin A.

Q I am a vegetarian— how can I increase my intake of omega-3 fats?

If you don't want to eat oily fish, try walnuts, flaxseeds, and flaxseed oil, otherwise known as linseed oil, for your omega-3 fats. These foods contain the short-chain omega-3 fats that have to be converted to long-chain fats in your body. Linseeds can be added to breakfast cereals or salads or you could also take supplements that contain flaxseed oil.

Q I think dairy foods make my arthritis worse. If I cut them out of my diet how can I get enough calcium?

If you can't eat dairy products then good sources of calcium include certain dried fruits (figs), green leafy vegetables (spinach, kale, and spring greens), legumes, almonds and Brazil nuts, sesame seeds, and fish such as sardines or whitebait (including the bones). Soy and rice milk *with added calcium* are suitable alternatives to cow's milk. Most varieties are fortified with calcium now—check the label. Other soy products, such as tofu, are rich in calcium.

Q I don't really like many fruits or vegetables—how can I make the most of the vitamins and minerals in them?

Eat them when they are really fresh. Eat vegetables raw or cook them as soon as possible after buying. If you're not using peeled or chopped fruits or vegetables right away, cover and chill them. Cook fruits and vegetables in as little water as possible, then retain the water to use in soups, casseroles, stews, and sauces. Don't soak or overcook them as vitamins and minerals can be lost.

Q What are antioxidants and are they beneficial for people with arthritis?

Antioxidants are nutrients that neutralize substances called free radicals, which help defend us against bacteria and other harmful particles, but can damage cells when they accumulate. Antioxidants include vitamins C (found in citrus fruits, berries, and green vegetables) and E (found in wheatgerm, vegetable oils, nuts, and seeds), beta-carotene (found in red and orange fruits and vegetables), and the trace mineral selenium (found in Brazil nuts). Preliminary research has shown that green tea, which is rich in antioxidants, may help people with osteoarthritis. Antioxidants are good for everybody and are especially important if you have arthritis or want to prevent it.

Q Are some fruit and vegetables better than others?

All fruits and vegetables are good sources of nutrients but some are better than others because they are particularly good sources of vitamins, minerals, and antioxidants. Most brightly colored fruits and vegetables contain antioxidants. Bananas, mushrooms, and tomatoes are good sources of potassium, a mineral that helps muscles work properly and contributes to maintaining healthy bones. Some prescribed drugs for arthritis can lower the level of potassium in the blood, which can be prevented by including potassium-rich foods in the diet.

Q Arthritis makes me feel so tired most of the time. What can I eat to give me an energy boost?

Some nutritious snacks, such as bananas or dried fruits, between meals can help give you that boost of energy. Or try a handful or two of nuts and raisins or crackers with peanut butter or honey—or both if you like. If your appetite is good you could have a bowl of breakfast cereal and cold milk. Avoid too many sugary snacks—they may give you a quick buzz of energy but it won't last long.

Q Is it true that folic acid can relieve the side effects of some arthritis drugs?

Yes. Folic acid (also called folate) can help alleviate the side effects of some of the medications for rheumatoid arthritis, such as methotrexate and sulfasalazine (see p92). To counteract these side effects, a high dose of folic acid (1–5mg) is usually prescribed once a week, or a lower dose taken daily. You can also boost your natural intake of folic acid by eating a whole range of foods. These include green leafy vegetables (such as cabbage, spinach, and brussels sprouts), beans, whole grains, wholegrain bread, fortified breakfast cereals, liver, yeast extract, egg yolk, as well as milk and other dairy products.

Avoiding foods

Q Do I need to eliminate any foods from my diet?

Many unsubstantiated claims have been made for the benefits of eliminating specific foods, or food groups, or of focusing on so-called "superfoods" to reduce the pain and inflammation of arthritis. It is important that you regard these claims with extreme caution. Dietitians and doctors generally do not recommend such diets because they could be detrimental to your general health and may even deprive your body of essential nutrients just when you need them most. If you do want to explore the possibilities of special diets, consult a registered dietitian first. For more information, contact the American Dietetic Association.

Q I've been avoiding certain foods for 6 months now and am not sure it's helping. How can I tell if this elimination diet works?

If you're not sure that avoiding the foods has helped, try adding them back into your diet one at a time—say one food each week. Keep a diary of the different foods you eat each day and make a note of any symptoms that you feel. This way you may be able to tell if any of the foods are making you feel worse. If so, then continue to avoid that food but otherwise put the others back into your diet and enjoy eating them.

Q Should I avoid cow's milk protein and drink soy milk instead?

There is no need to avoid cow's milk because of the protein content—if you do so you will reduce your intake of calcium, which is vital for maintaining strong, healthy bones. Soy milk does not contain calcium unless the manufacturer has added it. If you continue to drink soy milk, make sure that you buy one that has been fortified with calcium.

Myth "Food sensitivity plays a major role in provoking arthritic symptoms"

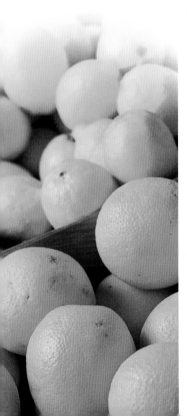

Truth Most inflammation is not caused by sensitivity to one particular food or another, although some people do find that certain foods worsen their symptoms. It is better to follow a diet containing foods that are good for your health and may help lessen inflammation, rather than to focus on potential dietary culprits. Ask your healthcare provider to refer you to a registered dietitian if you feel you are sensitive toward certain foods.

Q Will cutting down on purine-rich foods keep my gout at bay?

If you are prone to repeated attacks of gout, or your symptoms are not adequately controlled by medication (see p36), then avoiding purine-rich foods may help you minimize acute attacks. Many foods are rich in purines, which can cause an increase in uric acid levels when broken down in the body during digestion. These purine-rich foods include organ meats (liver, kidneys, and heart); wild game (such as venison, grouse, and duck); some oil-rich fish (such as mackerel, herring, shellfish, and anchovies); yeast (extract and tablets); and hard, extra mature cheese. Beer is particularly high in purines, and all alcoholic beverages are high in calories, so restrict how much you drink—or better yet, cut out alcohol altogether. Drinking plenty of water will prevent dehydration and further reduce the risk of gout attacks.

Q We are always being told to eat oily fish, but now I've got gout I've been advised not to eat it. What should I do?

Unfortunately, many purine-rich foods are also highly nutritious; some, such as oil-rich fish, are particularly recommended for inflammatory conditions such as rheumatoid arthritis. Try eating a little oily fish and boost your omega-3 fat intake by eating walnuts and linseeds (in cereals and salads) or by taking flaxseed supplements (see p153).

Q Should I avoid eating oranges and tomatoes because of the risk that the acid will cause my rheumatoid arthritis to flare up?

Many people who have rheumatoid arthritis believe that citrus fruits and tomatoes may cause their joints to become inflamed. However, there really is no evidence that avoiding these foods is beneficial for people with rheumatoid arthritis. What you do miss out on are delicious foods that are valuable sources of vitamin C as well as folic acid.

Weight control

Q What is the body mass index index (BMI)?

Body mass index (BMI) is the relationship of your weight in kilograms divided by the square of your height in meters. In pounds and inches, the calculation is more difficult: divide your weight in pounds by the square of your height in inches, then multiply by 703. For example, a man who weighs 220lb (100kg) and is 71in (1.8m) tall has a BMI of 31. A woman who weighs 154lb (70kg) and is 63in (1.6m) tall has a BMI of 27. Your BMI will fall into one of 4 groups: underweight (BMI of less than 18.5); healthy weight (BMI of 18.5–24.9); overweight (BMI of 25–29.9); and obese (BMI of 30 or above). This advice is for adults, not children.

Q Why is BMI so important?

One of the most important things you can do is to keep your weight within a healthy range. Being either too fat or too thin not only affects how well you manage your arthritis but also affects other aspects of your health.

Q I have been obese for some time—why is it so important that I lose weight now that I have developed arthritis?

Losing excess weight will help you keep active, which is important in maintaining joint health. If you are overweight it could make your arthritis worse, since you will be putting extra stress on your joints, particularly your hips and knees. Excess fat is also thought to be directly linked to the process of inflammation, so people with rheumatoid arthritis should be especially careful. Besides affecting the symptoms of arthritis, carrying excess weight puts an additional strain on your heart and is a major risk factor for serious disorders such as stroke, high blood pressure (hypertension), and diabetes.

Q **Are there any simple tips to help me lose weight?**

Keep a food and activity diary for a couple of weeks to get a true picture of your eating and activity habits. Then think of ways to improve them. Try to lose weight steadily and don't skip meals, especially breakfast. Serve food on smaller plates and try to eat more slowly—take your time and enjoy the taste of your food. If you're hungry between meals, drink a large glass of water. Choose non-fat dairy products, cut down on alcohol, and avoid sweetened soft drinks. Snack on fruit and raw vegetables, not cookies and candy. Stay active.

Q **I'm really quite skinny—should I put on weight now that I have been diagnosed with rheumatoid arthritis?**

Not necessarily. If "skinny" is normal for you, then putting on weight may not help. If you have lost weight because you've been unwell then yes, it would help to regain your body weight. Putting on weight can sometimes be harder than trying to lose it. If you're unsure about what to eat, ask your doctor to refer you to a registered dietitian.

Q **Are there any simple tips to help me put on weight?**

Eating to gain weight may add unhealthy levels of fat to your diet, especially if you use full-fat dairy products. Check with your doctor or dietitian before increasing your intake of fats and oils or taking up any of the following suggestions. Eat several small meals during the day, rather than attempting (and failing) to eat one or two large ones. Try milkshakes made with fruit or soups with added milk or cream. Eat nutritious snacks between meals, such as cheese, peanut butter, and dried fruits. You can also include fish or lean meat in your diet every day to boost your protein intake. Add butter or cheese sauces to vegetables. A small glass of sherry or ale might perk up your appetite before a meal.

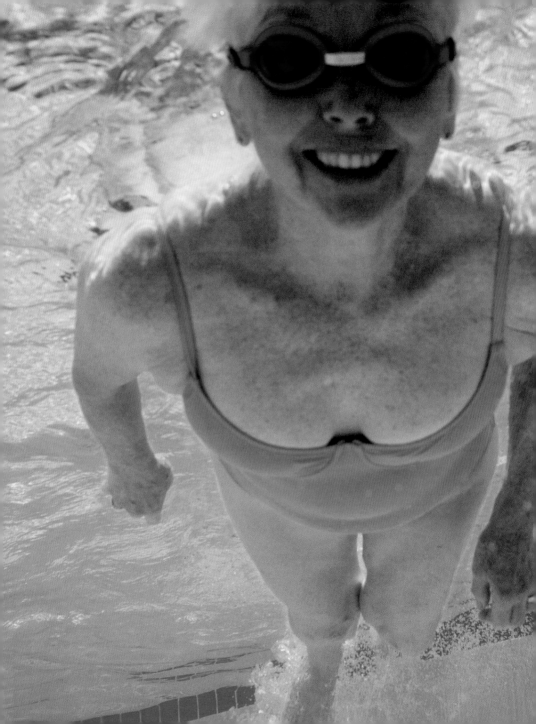

Physical activity

Exercise is known to be very effective in reducing joint pain and disability, yet few people with arthritis receive good advice about it. It may seem like a paradox, but simple physical activities—not rest—can not only keep your joints and muscles working well together but can also help reduce pain and disability.

Getting enough exercise

Q How can physical activity and exercise be good for me now that several of my joints are affected by arthritis?

Movement is good for your joints. Exercise and regular physical activity will ensure that your joints and muscles work effectively by making them do what they were designed to do—move, contract, and work. An increasing amount of evidence indicates that exercise has many benefits for people with arthritis. It reduces pain, improves muscle strength, and makes you feel less tired. It can also help restore and maintain mobility (see p171), as well as strengthen bones, improve breathing and circulation, reduce stress, stimulate digestion, keep body weight down, and encourage better sleep patterns.

Q Why can't I rely on other treatments, such as drugs, to relieve my symptoms?

Many people with arthritis do not realize the benefits of exercise and rely on other treatments, particularly drugs, to help them. Although anti-inflammatory and analgesic drugs can reduce some of the symptoms of arthritis, such as inflammation and pain, they do not alter the underlying condition, or prevent the problems that arthritis can cause, including joint damage, weakness, fatigue, and disability. Some drugs can have unpleasant side effects in certain people. Exercise may help you reduce arthritis symptoms.

Q What happens to my muscles and joints if I don't exercise them regularly?

Anyone who stops being active for a prolonged period of time will find that their muscles and bones grow weaker and the cartilage lining their joints becomes thinner. As a result, they feel tired sooner and their joints will stiffen up. In fact, inactivity is bad for your joints. It causes both stiffness and muscle weakness, which accelerate joint damage, leading to greater pain and disability.

Q **Is it true that if I don't exercise and remain inactive I will almost certainly develop health problems?**

Yes. It is difficult to predict exactly what those health problems will be because they vary from one person to another. Exercise and physical activity help your heart, lungs, and blood vessels become stronger and more efficient, so that you can do more with less effort. Other benefits include less cholesterol, better control of diabetes, protection from some forms of cancer, less depression, increased self-confidence, and greater dignity, independence, and self-esteem.

TEN EXERCISE RULES

1. While exercising, always ensure that you are stable and safe. For example, if you stand, have something near to hold on to.
2. Start each new exercise gently and cautiously.
3. Increase the amount or kind of exercise gradually over a period of days and weeks.
4. Rest on "bad" days when joints are feeling painful or inflamed. When the pain subsides, resume gently.
5. Exercise regularly but avoid causing prolonged pain or discomfort.
6. Exercise using controlled movement; quality is as important as quantity.
7. Set yourself realistic goals.
8. Write an action plan and tell people your goals.
9. Pace yourself—little and often is just as good as one strenuous session.
10. Understand that exercise does not cure arthritis and episodes of pain are usually not related to exercising.

Myth "To be effective, exercise must be strenuous"

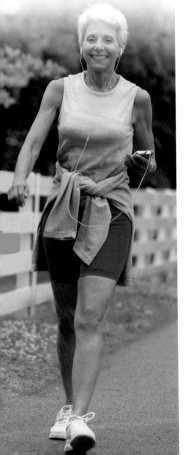

Truth Doing almost any physical activity regularly is better than doing nothing regularly. On the whole, the more you do the better, but it doesn't have to be hard work. Acquiring the full health benefits from exercise does undeniably require effort, determination, and willpower. But it does not require bouts of exhausting, strenuous exercise, nor do you need a personal trainer, health club, or expensive equipment and facilities.

Q **Can people with inflammatory arthritis exercise without any problems?**

Yes. An inflammatory arthritis, such as rheumatoid arthritis, doesn't prevent you from exercising. In fact, exercise and movement are important in managing ankylosing spondylitis to prevent the condition from getting worse. Always discuss your exercise needs with an experienced healthcare professional—your doctor or physical therapist. Don't exercise during periods of joint pain and inflammation, but start again when things have settled.

Q **Will I be able to cut down on the medication for my arthritis if I exercise regularly?**

If you have inflammatory arthritis, such as rheumatoid arthritis, continue your prescribed medicine and discuss your exercise needs with your doctor. If you have osteoarthritis, ask your doctor if you can reduce the dosage you need to control your symptoms. You may take it when you need it to give you most relief, such as before going out, going to bed, or before exercise. Medication can make your life more comfortable and bearable, and allow you to be physically active. Drugs and exercise can help separately; together, they can be very effective. If you start exercising, you are likely to experience episodes of pain, which may not be as often, or as bad, or last as long.

Q **I don't really want to go to a gym or special classes—can I just exercise on my own?**

Exercise does not have to mean going to a health club. Most activities that you do in your daily life are "informal" and therefore have the same potential health benefits as formal exercise. These include walking (see p168), gardening, shopping, doing housework, or spending a day outdoors. The important thing is to find an activity you want to do that is enjoyable, affordable, and available. You need to feel comfortable doing it; then find the exercise level that is right for you and aim to maintain it. If you don't, you will probably soon stop.

Q **I go walking every day—does this count as good exercise?**

Walking is a very good example of a simple but effective informal exercise that is easy to do on your own without specialist equipment or facilities. In fact, for people with arthritis, walking is one of the best and most pleasurable ways to exercise. Walking is not too stressful or exhausting—simply walk regularly and comfortably at your own chosen pace.

Q **Are there any tips for safe and enjoyable walking?**

People with arthritis often find that walking increases their pain and this can cause a concern. First of all, make sure you are wearing good, supportive shoes or boots. If walking is painful, avoid long walks because they only make the pain worse. See how far you can walk before the pain starts and walk little and often within this distance at a comfortable pace. Rest if you need to. A walking stick may help you walk further. Each week, increase the distance a little. Vary your walks to make them interesting and enjoyable.

Q **How can I tell if I have done too much exercise?**

It is not unusual to experience muscle ache, tenderness, and stiffness after doing a new activity. This discomfort may increase for a day or so, but then should gradually ease. If the discomfort or pain lasts for more than 3 days, wakes you at night, or if your joints feel hot and swollen, you have probably been overexuberant and done too much. Reduce the amount of exercise you are doing for a couple of days to allow things to settle and omit any exercise you think may have caused the problems—you might add them later, very gradually and slowly. If unpleasant symptoms persist use simple ways to relieve pain, such as hot or cold packs (see p138), but if they continue, see your doctor.

Q **I'm not sure how to start an exercise program—are there some simple tips that would help me?**

Don't be too ambitious at the start. If you are not normally active, begin with gentle exercises that are not weight-bearing—for example, slowly bend and straighten your knees as you sit on a bed, sofa, or on the floor. Over the following days, weeks, or even months, gradually increase the frequency and intensity of these exercises. Try to exercise for about 30 minutes on most days of the week. It doesn't have to be all at once—you could break it up into two 15-minute or three 10-minute periods. Doing a little physical activity regularly is better than doing none at all. Within reason, the more you do the better. Remember, every little bit will help you.

Q **What is my eventual aim with my exercise program?**

Your eventual aim is to do weight-bearing exercises or activities that use your body weight as a resistance. Examples of these are stepping on and off a low step (see p174) or standing up after sitting in a low chair. Whatever exercise or activity you do, be sure to pace yourself, balancing the activity with rest.

Q **I'm not very good at motivating myself—how can I motivate myself to keep going?**

Get your family and friends to support you. Monitor yourself—keep account of how well you have done. Believe in yourself and your ability to be active. Exercise for the right reasons—because it helps you, you want to, and you enjoy it. Think about how to overcome barriers and how to get around them. Lack of time, pain, or bad weather may be a genuine reason why you cannot exercise, but don't use them as an excuse. Plan for a relapse—when the going gets tough, decide how you are going to "tough" it out and resume your exercises. Reward yourself when you achieve a goal.

GOAL SETTING AND ACTION PLANS

Setting goals and making action plans can help you with the level and amount of exercise and physical activity you want to achieve. Consider your current level of activity and the impact arthritis is having on your daily life. Ask yourself what activities you would like to perform more easily if you could.

- Initially, set yourself simple, challenging, but realistic goals that you can achieve within a few days or a week—and pursue them in a very focused way.

- Decide exactly what you are going to do—and when, where, and how you are going to do it. Write this out in a formal action plan, pin it up on the wall where you can see it every day—and stick to it.

- Tell your family, friends, and colleagues about your action plan. They can remind you to do things and can become a tremendous source of encouragement, support, and motivation.

- Monitor your progress. Circle on a calendar the days when you have exercised—and aim to cover it with circles. When you have achieved a goal, tell everybody and reward yourself with something you like.

- If you want, revise your goals by making those you have achieved slightly more challenging so that you are always pushing the boundaries of what you do. With a little more effort you will be amazed at how much more you can do for yourself, how much easier life becomes, and how much better you will feel about yourself.

- If you can't achieve a goal, don't worry about it. Reassess the goal and aim for something less ambitious and slightly easier.

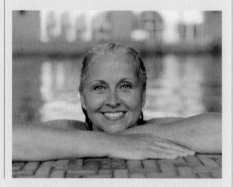

Maintaining mobility

Q I don't seem to be getting anywhere fast and I'm tempted to give up. Can you recommend any particular exercises to maintain mobility?

Although your temptation is understandable, it would be a mistake because you would start to lose your mobility and your flexibility. There are a number of exercise sequences you can do for different body parts. These include exercises for your neck (see Head turns and Head rolls, pp172–173), shoulders, back, and legs and hips (see Step-ups, Gentle squats and Hip rotations, pp174–175). Always make sure you are stable and safe, exercise within your comfort zone, and stop at once if you feel dizzy.

Q What kind of exercises do I need to do?

Start with low-impact exercises that do not involve you bearing any weight. These are the ones in which you sit or lie on the floor or on a bed. Then build up to doing the weight-bearing exercises and functional activities, such as walking (see p168).

Q Can I adapt any type of exercise to suit my needs?

Yes, but within reason. Be careful if you are not used to exercising. What seems like a simple and easy task can cause discomfort and pain, which may lead to anxiety that you have caused damage by doing too much. Err on the side of caution—start gently and increase gradually. Once you feel comfortable doing an exercise, try to "nudge the boundaries" of your capabilities, challenging yourself to gently and gradually move a little further or work a little harder. Once you have reached a level you are content with, keep that level of exercise going to maintain the gains you have achieved. Performing the exercises well, with controlled movement, is as important as repeating the exercise more often or for longer.

Neck exercises

Head turns and head rolls are simple neck exercises that you can practice regularly to improve the movement of your head on your shoulders. Before you start, make sure you are standing—or sitting—straight and tall. Imagine a string, connected to the crown at the top of your head, is holding you up and extending your neck. Keep your shoulders and upper limbs relaxed at all times. Breathe in through your nose and out through your mouth, slowly and gently.

HEAD TURNS

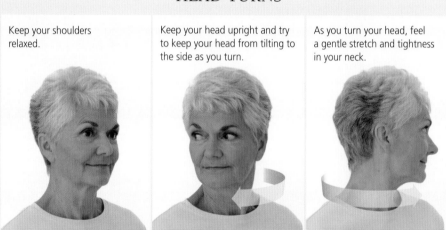

Keep your shoulders relaxed.

Keep your head upright and try to keep your head from tilting to the side as you turn.

As you turn your head, feel a gentle stretch and tightness in your neck.

You can do this head-turning exercise either sitting or standing. If you are standing, make sure you are next to a wall or something to grab on to just in case you feel dizzy.

Slowly turn your head to look over your right shoulder without tilting it to the side. Feel a gentle stretch and tightness in your neck. Breathe gently. Hold the position for 5 or 6 seconds.

Now turn to look over your left shoulder, again without tilting your head to the side. Hold the position for 5 or 6 seconds. Repeat the full exercise sequence another 5 or 6 times.

HEAD ROLLS

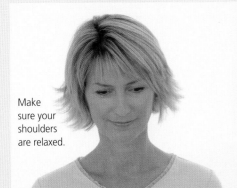

Make sure your shoulders are relaxed.

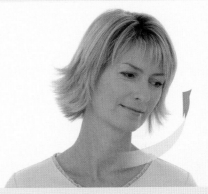

Start with your shoulders relaxed and your eyes looking forward. Slowly let your head fall to the front so that your chin drops down toward your chest and you are looking at the floor.

Slowly roll your head to the left. As you do so, bring your left ear as close to your left shoulder as you comfortably can, with your eyes looking in the direction your head is moving.

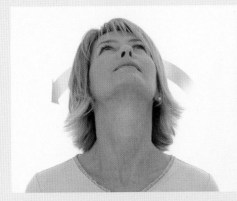

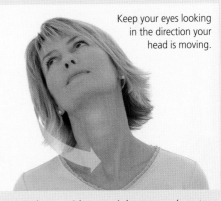

Keep your eyes looking in the direction your head is moving.

Continue to move your head in a wide circle, from left to right. When you reach midway, look upward toward the ceiling and feel a gentle stretch in the muscles in the front of your neck.

Come down with your right ear as close to your right shoulder as you comfortably can. Relax. Repeat 3 or 4 circles. Repeat the whole sequence, this time circling to the right.

Leg and hip exercises

The following exercises will help improve and maintain the mobility in your hips and knees. They help ease any stiffness you might feel and build up strength in the muscles surrounding the joints. People with arthritis of the knee or hip should find particular benefit from the step-ups. Make sure you always work within your comfort zone and avoid overextending yourself.

STEP-UPS

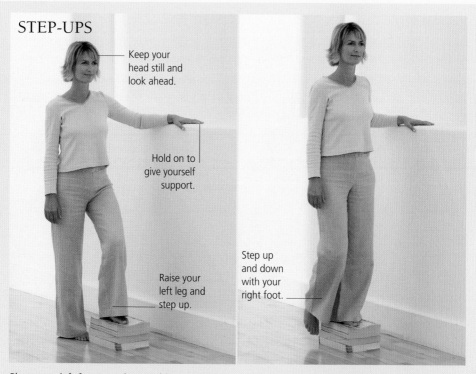

Keep your head still and look ahead.

Hold on to give yourself support.

Step up and down with your right foot.

Raise your left leg and step up.

Place your left foot on a low, stable step. Hold on to the wall, banisters, or chair for support. Step up and down with your right foot for a minute. Repeat 5 or 6 times. Repeat the exercise with your right foot on the step. As you gradually increase the number of step-ups, raise the height of the step (ensuring you are stable and safe) to a maximum of 18in (45cm).

GENTLE SQUATS

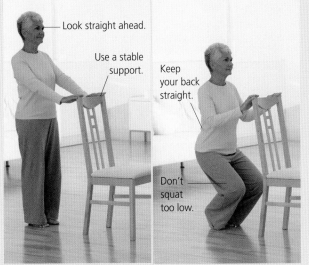

Look straight ahead.

Use a stable support.

Keep your back straight.

Don't squat too low.

Stand upright with your feet flat on the floor. Steady yourself by resting your hands on a stable object such as the back of a chair. Keeping your back straight, slowly bend your knees into a gentle squat and then straighten your knees until you are standing. Repeat 10 times. As you improve, squat down a little further, but not beyond 90 degrees, and never fully, which puts great strain on your knees.

HIP ROTATIONS

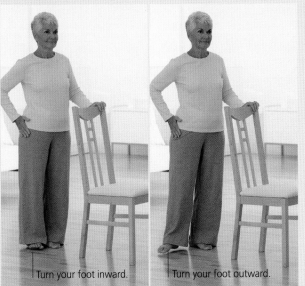

Turn your foot inward.

Turn your foot outward.

Stand upright with your left hand resting on a stable object, such as the back of a chair. Put your right hand on your right hip and raise the hip so your right foot is 1–1.5in (2–3cm) off the ground. Turn your foot to the left as far as possible (feel your hip turning inward under your hand). Hold the position for 5 or 6 seconds. Turn your foot out to the right and hold for 5 or 6 seconds. Repeat sequence 10 times, each side.

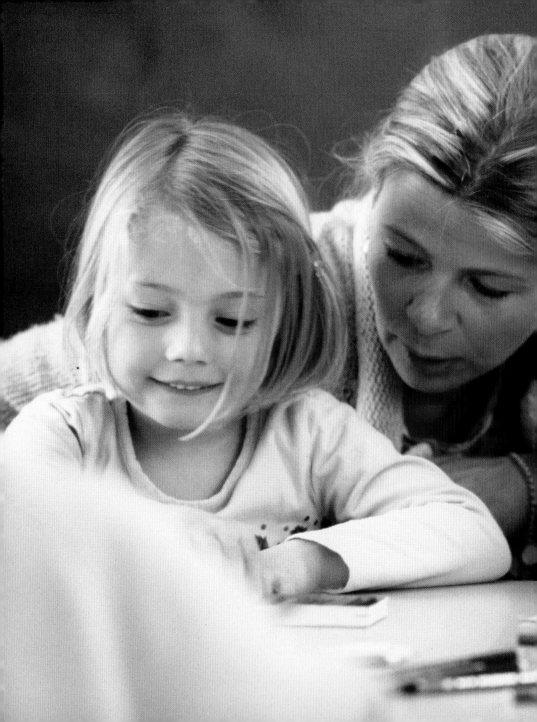

Children
with arthritis

Arthritis can be hard to detect in
children but often develops in a
similar way to arthritis in adults.
It may take months or years to
confirm a diagnosis of arthritis
in a child, let alone start effective
treatment. However, children with
arthritis can benefit from all kinds
of therapeutic care and support,
while at the same time receiving
help for their special needs—at
school, at home, and at play.

Understanding juvenile arthritis

Q How common is arthritis in children?

It is not common at all. Each year, arthritis affects about 1 child in every 1,000. Most cases of arthritis in children are mild and self-limiting. More severe types of arthritis affect approximately 1 child in every 10,000.

Q What is juvenile arthritis?

Most of the arthritis in children is due to a group of inflammatory disorders known as juvenile arthritis. Also known as juvenile idiopathic arthritis or juvenile rheumatoid arthritis, it involves pain, inflammation, and swelling in at least one joint. It may run in families and seems to result from an abnormal response of the immune system. There are 5 main types, depending on the joints involved in the early months of disease and the involvement of other organs. In oligoarthritis, for instance, which accounts for about half of the cases of juvenile arthritis, fewer than 4 joints are involved.

Q If my child experiences pain in one or more joints does it mean she has juvenile arthritis?

Joint pains are common and only rarely indicate a serious condition is present. There is a small chance they might be due to arthritis, other serious musculoskeletal problems, or a chronic pain syndrome of unknown cause such as fibromyalgia (see p43). Other causes, which are also uncommon, include inherited disorders of the protein collagen and other connective tissue components, and blood problems, such as sickle cell disease. Pain can also be due to other minor musculoskeletal complaints.

Q **What are the signs that my child might be affected by juvenile arthritis?**

Arthritis may be hard to diagnose in a child and the first features can be nonspecific, such as pain or general illness. Arthritis changes the way a child walks or uses his or her arms, legs, hands, and feet. Pain often limits the movement of an affected joint, although younger children will not always complain of pain. If the legs are involved the child may start to limp or walk with difficulty. Another sign to look for is swelling in a child's joint, especially if accompanied by pain and stiffness that persists, or is worse in the morning or after a nap.

Q **Can children with juvenile arthritis develop osteoporosis?**

Yes. Children who have been badly affected by juvenile arthritis can later develop osteoporosis, in which bones lose their density and become weak and porous. If doctors are concerned, they may use scans called DXA (dual energy X-ray absorptiometry) to identify it early. Treatment may involve bisphosphonate drugs and, if the child is treated with corticosteroids, calcium and. Vitamin D supplements may be prescribed, too.

Q **Will blood tests reveal whether my child has juvenile arthritis?**

Just as with adults, a positive result for any blood test (see p61) does not necessarily confirm that your child has arthritis. Nevertheless, the presence of either antinuclear antibodies or rheumatoid factor (see p62) is highly suggestive of juvenile arthritis. About 1 in 4 children with arthritis, particularly oligoarthritis, test positive for antinuclear antibodies. Rheumatoid factor usually indicates polyarthritis—a type of juvenile arthritis involving at least 5 joints that will continue into adult life. Children with systemic arthritis, in which the internal organs may be affected, and polyarthritis invariably have a high ESR reading (see p60).

Myth "Children are never affected by arthritis"

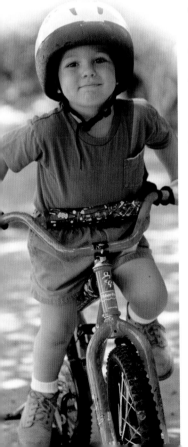

Truth Few people realize that arthritis affects children as well as adults, even though this is uncommon. In fact, juvenile arthritis usually seems to catch everyone by surprise, probably because it is easy to overlook and difficult to diagnose. It may take months or years for doctors and pediatric rheumatologists to confirm a diagnosis of arthritis in a child, let alone start effective treatment.

Q Will my child need an X-ray or MRI scan?

To help confirm a diagnosis or assess the severity of arthritis, your child may need an X–ray or, rarely, a magnetic resonance imaging (MRI) scan to show the extent of joint damage. They can identify the presence of bone erosion in one or more joints or show the presence of excessive fluid within a joint.

Q If my child is diagnosed with arthritis, what sort of healthcare will she be given?

In some areas your child will be looked after by a pediatric rheumatologist (a pediatrician specially trained in managing arthritis). In other areas, the role is shared between an adult rheumatologist and a general pediatrician, supported by physical therapists and occupational therapists. The main goal of this care team is to manage arthritis while keeping the child in good physical condition and an active part of your family and community. Your child is treated to reduce swelling and pain, and is encouraged to exercise to maintain muscle tone and movement in the affected joints.

Q What drugs will my child need to take?

Your child's doctor can prescribe NSAIDs (see p83), such as ibuprofen and naproxen. Children are not usually treated with aspirin because of the potential side effects. The same DMARDs are used in children as are used in adults (see p92). Methotrexate is preferred because the small doses needed to relieve symptoms do not usually cause potentially dangerous side effects. When a child's arthritis is severe and uncontrolled, or when the inflammation affects internal organs, rheumatologists may add steroids (see p87) such as prednisone to existing treatments for a short period. Biologic agents (see p93) may be prescribed for children with polyarthritis who have gained little relief from other drugs.

Special needs

Q Will my child's arthritis prevent her from going to school?

No, not unless it is very severe. However, life at school can be made a little easier. Helping your child conserve energy is vital: take her to school in the morning when joint stiffness can be acute; keep textbooks at home so she doesn't have to carry heavy bags; if possible arrange for lessons to be held on the ground floor to avoid stairs and the rush between classes. Arthritis in the hands and wrists can make writing hard, slow, or painful: let your child use pens with special grips (see p124), take breaks from writing, wear a wrist splint, and use a computer keyboard whenever possible.

Q I'm afraid that my child will lose out on the benefits of play. How can she join in more and take part in active play?

Play is an essential part of growing up. With some creativity and a little ingenuity, it is possible to persuade every child with arthritis to be actively engaged in play. Your child needs to be careful with exercise choices. For instance, it is best to avoid contact sports and activities that will overuse one part of the body. It is also important to avoid activities that stress those joints that are inflamed. However, it is also essential to encourage activities that keep children together with their friends.

Q My youngest child has just been diagnosed with juvenile arthritis. How can we as parents encourage a normal family life?

Try to make adjustments and contingency plans, particularly on days when the arthritis is bad. The family needs to accept all the uncertainties with equanimity, and to encourage ideas for activities on active days as well as quiet ones. Vitally important, too, is the need to explain to the child that getting arthritis is nobody's fault. Joining a support group can help.

Long-term outlook

Q **What is the long-term outlook for a child with arthritis?**

Overall, the prognosis for juvenile arthritis is relatively good. With modern treatments and management techniques, most children do very well. However, some types of arthritis that involve many joints or have many systemic symptoms can pose problems in the long term.

Q **Will my child's arthritis affect her growth?**

Many children with juvenile chronic arthritis, especially those with systemic polyarthritis, do not grow normally. One typical feature is a small lower jaw and a small chin. The main causes of affected growth are chronic inflammation, corticosteroid treatment, and poor nutrition. However, active treatment and minimal doses of steroids can help reduce the degree of retarded growth. Prolonged inflammation can make it difficult to bend and straighten the knees, and may damage the small joints of the hand, even the neck joints. Orthopedic surgeons have developed techniques to replace a joint that fails, release a joint that cannot straighten properly, and remove excessive cartilage from a joint.

Q **Are there any serious complications that my child may develop in the future?**

Some children with arthritis can develop serious organ problems, either due to the disease or its treatment with drugs. Problems include an inflamed pericardium (the membrane around the heart) and kidney failure. Inflammation of the blood vessels can affect many different organs, too. Uveitis, in which the uvea layer of the eye becomes inflamed, is potentially debilitating and can result in blindness. However, expert care and monitoring from eye surgeons can minimize the risks.

Useful addresses

Arthritis Foundation
1330 West Peachtree Street, Ste. 100
Atlanta, GA 30309
Tel: (800) 568-4045
Tel: (404) 872-7100
Email: help@arthritis.org
Website: www.arthritis. org
The Arthritis Foundation has 46
local offices around the US. Enter
your zip code on the AF website to
locate the office nearest you. Each
local office has a toll-free help line
and information on local programs,
services, and events. There is also a
physician referral for each region.

**American Association of
Orthopaedic Medicine**
600 Pembrook Drive
Woodland Park, CO 80863
Tel: (800) 992-2063
Email: aaom@aaomed.org
Website: www.aom.org

**American Academy of Physical
Medicine and Rehabilitation**
330 North Wabash Avenue, Ste. 2500
Chicago, IL 60611
Tel: (312-464-9700
Email: info@aapmr.org
Website: www.aapmr.org

American College of Rheumatology
1800 Century Place
Atlanta, GA 30345
Tel: (404) 633-3777
Email: acr@rheumatology.org
Website: www.rheumatology.org

**American Autoimmune Related
Diseases Association**
22100 Gratiot Avenue
East Detroit, MI 48021
Tel: (586) 776-3900
Website: www.aarda.org

**American Occupational Therapy
Assocation**
4720 Montgomery Lane
PO Box 31220
Bethesda, MD 20824
Tel: (301) 652-2682
Tel: (800) 377-8555 (TDD)
Website: www.aota.org

The Arthritis Society of Canada
393 University Avenue, Ste. 1700
Toronto, Ontario M5G 1E6
Canada
Tel: (800) 321-1433
Tel: (416) 979-7228
Email: info@arthritis.ca
Website: www.arthritis.ca

Index

A

abatacept 93
ABCDE method 142–3
abnormal immune response 42
acetabulum 21
acetaminophen 83–4
action plans 170
acupuncture 71
alcohol 149, 159
Alexander technique 75
allopurinol 36
American Academy of Orthopedic
  Surgery 100
American Association of Psychotherapists 67
American Dietetic Association 157
Americans with Disabilities Act (1990)
  117, 131
    Accessibility Guidelines for
    Buildings and Facilities Act 117, 131
analgesics 83, 88, 90
anesthesia 106
ankylosing spondylitis 32–3, 48
    features 33
    joints affected 32
    long-term outlook 33
    mobility 33
    treatment 33
antinuclear antibodies 62, 179
antioxidants 151, 155–6
ANTs (automatic negative thoughts)
  141

applying heat or cold 138
aquatherapy 137
Arthritis Foundation 67, 105, 124,
  129–30
arthroplasty see joint replacement
arthroscopy 62
artificial implants 103
artificial joint 103, 113
aspirin 83
assistive devices 119, 122–7
autoantibodies 61
autoimmune disorder 53
avoiding injuries 19
avranofin 93
azathioprine 41, 92

B

back pain 48–9
bendrofluazide 35
biologic agents 29, 53, 90–1, 93,
  181
biomechanics 133
blood clots 111–2
blood tests 60–2
    different types 61
body mass index (BMI) 160
bursitis 50
butterfly rash 40

C

C-reactive protein 60
calcium 155

calcium pyrophosphate dihydrate 37
canola oil 147
carbohydrates 146
caring for children 128–9
carpal tunnel syndrome 39, 51–2
cartilage 14, 16, 20
cartilage removal 21
causes of arthritis 10
celecoxib 86
children with arthritis 177
  long-term outlook 183
  special needs 182
chondroitin 23, 152–3
chondroplasty 99
citrus fruits 159
cod liver oil 153–4
codeine 83
colchicine 36
complementary therapies 70–1, 76–7
  herbal remedies 71
  practitioners 70
computerized tomography 59
connective tissues 9
connective tissue arthritis 9
cooking 122–3
corticosteroids 36–7, 47, 87, 90
counseling 67
COX-1 inhibitors 86
COX-2 inhibitors 86
cyclophosphamide 41
cyclosporin 41, 93

D

dairy products 155
Department of Veterans Affairs 131
depression 11, 28
DEXA 59, 179
diagnosis 57–9
  assessment 59
  examination 59
  medical history 59
  symptoms 58
diclofenac 84, 181
diet 66, 145–61
  avoiding foods 157–9
  nutrients 151–6
  supplements 152–3
  weight control 160–1
  well-balanced 146–9
Disabled Parking placard 131
Disability Employment Agency (DEA) 117–8
DMARDs 29–30, 33, 53, 90–3, 181
  commonly prescribed 92–3
  during pregnancy 91
domestic activities 120–7
driving 130–1
drugs 68, 79–91, 164
  generic 68
  online purchase 68
  side effects 81
drug safety 80–1

E

ECG 105
emotional changes 140, 142
encephalins 136

endorphins 71, 136
ergonomics 133
ESR test 60
essential oils 76
estrogen 20
etoricoxib 86
exercise 31, 116, 136, 163, 164–75

F

family life 128–9
fatigue 11–2
FDA (Food and Drug Administration)
    86
fibromyalgia 9, 43–5, 178
    exercise 45
    symptoms 45
    tender points 44
    treatment 45
fibrous tissue 14
fish oils 152–3
flaxseed oil 153–4
fluids 149
folic acid 156, 159
footwear 130

G

gardening 122
giant cell arteritis 42
glucosamine 23, 88, 152–3
goal setting 170
gout 9, 34–6
    antihypertensive drugs 35
    cancer treatment 35
    diet 36, 159
    joints affected 35

gout cont.
    treatment 36
    triggers 34
    uric acid levels 35–6, 60
growth hormone 45

H

half-joint replacement 101
halibut liver oil 153
health care 57, 63, 66–7, 70–7
herbal medicines 71–3
    boswellia 73
    bromelain 73
    burdock 73
    cat's claw 72
    cayenne 72
    devil's claw 72
    ginger 73
    turmeric 73
hip replacement 100–103, 108–9
histamine 12
HLA-B27 32
HLA-DR4 27
homeopathy 75
housework 121–3
hyaluronic acid 87
hydrocodone 83
hydrotherapy 137
hydroxychloroquine 41, 91–2

I

ibuprofen 83–5, 152
imaging 59
immune system 12
implant dislocation 112–3

indomethacin 84
infections 54, 104, 111
infective arthritis 54–5
  treatment 55
inflammation 12, 20, 62, 71, 76, 90,
  128, 153, 160, 164
inflammatory arthritis 9, 16, 28, 50,
  53, 116
injectable gold 93
injury 12, 18–20
intra-articular injections 23, 87
isotope bone scans 59

J

joint 11, 13, 16–17
  failure of 13
  imaging 59
  infection 10
  inflammation 10, 12–3, 24–5, 32,
    53–4, 89–90, 116, 178–9, 183
  pain 10–13, 23, 39, 50, 54–5, 89,
    119, 132, 178
  protection 132–5
  replacement 100–101, 110, 112–3
  stiffness 10, 12–3, 22–3, 50, 54,
    75, 89
  surgery 29, 96–7
  surgical realignment see osteotomy
  swelling 10, 12–3, 23, 132, 178–9
  synovial 14
  tenderness 11
  types of 14–5
joint replacement surgery 59, 63,
  95–7, 102–3, 109
joint space 16

juvenile arthritis 178–83
  blood tests 179
  growth 183

K

ketoprofen 83–5
knee implant 102
knee replacement 101–2, 108–9
knee surgery 21

L

lateral epicondylitis see tennis elbow
leflunomide 92
leucocytes 27
lifestyle changes 115
lifting objects 135
linseed oil see flaxseed oil
localized soft-tissue disorders 47–50
loss of function 12
low-impact exercises 171
lower back pain 48–9
  treatment 49
lumiracoxib 86
lupus 9, 40–1
  areas affected 41
  risk factors 40
  symptoms 40–1
  treatment 41
lyme disease 54–5

M

massage 137
mast cells 12
Medicaid 131
Medicare 131

meditation 141
Mediterranean diet 151
menopause 20
methotrexate 61, 91–2, 181
minimally invasive surgery 98
mobility 109, 164, 171–5
motivation 169
movement therapies 75
MRI 59, 181
mycophenolate mofetil 41

N

naproxen 83–4, 181
natural remedies 74
natural remedies see complementary
  therapies
noninflammatory arthritis 9
nonopioids 83
NSAIDs 23, 29, 37, 53, 68, 80–1,
  83–6, 88–90, 153, 181

O

Occupational Safety and Health Act
  (1970) 117
occupational therapy 66, 105, 119
old age 13
oligoarthritis 178–9
olive oil 154
omega-3 fats 151, 154
opioids 83
orthopedic specialists 63
orthopedic surgery 96–7
osteoarthritis 9, 13, 16–23, 48, 63, 87,
  98, 100–1, 110, 132, 152, 167
  drug treatment 23, 88–9

osteoarthritis (cont.)
  joints affected 16–7
  mobility 23
  nodal 18, 23
  of the hands 21
  of the knees 21
  risk factors 18–9
  weather 22
osteophytes 16, 59
osteoporosis 26, 31, 87, 179
osteotomy 98–9

P

pain 11, 21, 34–6, 42–3, 52–3, 70–1,
  96–7, 119, 128, 132, 152, 164, 168
  coping with 124–5, 136–9, 163
pain clinics 67
pericardium, inflamed 183
physical activity 134–5, 139, 163–71
physical therapy 66
Pilates 75
piroxicam 85
plantar fasciitis 47
plant oils 154
polyarthritis 179
polymyalgia rheumatica 42, 87
postoperative care 107, 109, 111
posture 120–1, 134
potassium 156
prednisone 90, 181
progesterone 20
preoperative care 104–6
propoxyphene 83
prostaglandins 89
protein 147

pseudogout 37
  treatment 37
psoriatic arthritis 53
  affected joints 53
  treatment 53
purines 159

Q

Qi Gong 75

R

reactive arthritis 54
reflexology 76
relaxation exercises 136, 139
repetitive strain injury 51
replacement knee surgery 20
revision surgery 113
rheumatoid arthritis 9, 13, 17,
  24–31, 42, 62–3, 75, 87, 90–2,
  101, 110, 117, 132, 147, 150–1,
  154, 161
  age 26, 31
  diet 150, 159
  disability 25
  drug treatment 90–1
  exercise 167
  genes 27
  joints affected 17, 27
  long-term problems 31
  mobility 29
  nodules 28
  osteoporosis 26
  other diseases 31
  prevention 31
  progression 25

rheumatoid arthritis cont.
  risk factors 24
  symptoms 24, 30
  treatment 29–30
  in women 26
rheumatoid factor 60, 62, 179
rheumatologists 63
rifumaxib 93
rofecoxib 86

S

S-adenosyl-L-methionine 152–3
safflower oil 147
salt 149
sciatica 48
self-help strategies 69
self-perception 11
septic arthritis see infective
  arthritis
sexual relationships 129
shoulder replacement 101
sickle cell disease 178
slipped disk 48
Social Security Department 117
soft-tissue massage 76–7
solving everyday problems 123
spa therapy 137
specialist stores 124
spine 98
splint 123
sports 19–20
SSRIs (selective serotonin reuptake
  inhibitors) 45
steroids 87, 181
stress, coping with 140–3

sulfasalazine 91–2
support groups 67
surgical treatments 95–113
    options 96–9
Swedish massage 76–7
symptoms of arthritis 12
synovial cavity 14
synovial fluid 36, 62
synovial membrane 14, 24
synovial sheath 52
synovium 50
systemic lupus erythematosus
    see lupus
systemic polyarthritis 183

T

tai chi 70, 75
tendinitis 50
tennis elbow 46–7
tenosynovitis 50
TENS 139
thiazide diuretics 35
thought-and-symptom diary
    142–3
tick bite 55
tophi 36
topical agents 82
torn ligaments 9
tramadol 83
    with acetaminophen 83
trauma 20
traveling 130–1
treatment options 64–5
tuberculosis 55
types of arthritis 9, 39

U

ultrasound 59
understanding arthritis 10–3
    identifying symptoms 12
    key characteristics 10
    main challenges 10
unsaturated fat 147–8
uric acid levels 60
uveitis 183

V

valdecoxib 86
vasculitis 39
viral arthritis 54–5
vitamin A (retinol) 153
vitamin C 159

W

walking 168
walking aid 130
warfarin 73, 153
water therapy 137
weight-bearing exercises 169
wheelchairs 130
work 116–8

X

X-rays 59, 105, 181

Y

yoga 51, 70, 75

Arthitis Foundation

The Arthritis Foundation is the largest US not-for-profit organization for people with arthritis, with 650,000 members. It has more than 50 state branches and over 150 offices throughout the US. The individual state branches run exercise programs and advice hotlines, and provide lists of local special referral units. The Arthritis Foundation has published many books, brochures, and videos for people with arthritis and produces a bimonthly magazine.

About the Consultant

Robin K. Dore, MD is a clinical professor in medicine in the Division of Rheumatology at the David Geffen School of Medicine, University of California at Los Angeles, as well as a board-certified rheumatologist practicing in Anaheim, California.

About the Authors

David L Scott is Professor of Clinical Rheumatology, King's College Hospital, London. *Howard Bird* is Professor of Pharmacological Rheumatology, University of Leeds. *Mike Hurley* is Professor of Physical Therapy, King's College, London. *Andrew Hamer* is Consultant Orthopedic Surgeon, Northern General Hospital, Sheffield. *Alison Hammond* is a Senior Lecturer in Rheumatology, School of Health Professions, University of Brighton. *Dorothy Pattison* is Lecturer in Dietetics, University of Plymouth. *Caroline Green* is a freelance health and science writer with a special interest in arthritis and complementary therapies.

Picture credits

The publisher would like to thank the following for their kind permission to reproduce their photographs: (Key: a-above; b-below/bottom; c-centre; f-far; l-left; r-right; t-top)

2 Corbis: Simon Marcus. 6 Corbis: LWA-Dann Tardif (l). Getty Images: Iconica/Zia Soleil (r). 7 Corbis: Rolf Bruderer (l); photocuisine/Roulier/Turiot (c). 8 Getty Images: Denis Boissavy. 22 Getty Images: The Image Bank/Buzz Bailey. 28 Corbis: Jose Luis Pelaez, Inc.. 31 Getty Images: Altrendo. 38 Getty Images: Stone/Bruce Ayres. 46 Corbis: Michael Keller. 49 Alamy Images: Bubbles Photolibrary (tr); Marwood Jenkins (tl). 56 Corbis: LWA-Dann Tardif. 61 Science Photo Library: AJ Photo. 64 Corbis: Larry Williams. 65 Corbis: Tom Stewart (r). Masterfile: Jerzyworks (l). 69 Corbis: Allana Wesley White (l). Getty Images: Taxi/Frederic Lucano (c). Science Photo Library: Ian Hooten (r). 78 Corbis: Larry Williams. 82 Photolibrary. 85 Photolibrary: Workbook, Inc/Larry Williams. 94 Corbis: LWA-Dann Tardif. 97 Corbis: Helen King (r); Tom & Dee Ann McCarthy (l). 102 courtesy Mr AJ Hamer FRCS(Orth) , Northern General Hospital, Sheffield: (b). 103 Science Photo Library: Dr P. Marazzi (r). 108 Corbis: Rolf Bruderer. 110 Corbis: Roy McMahon. 114 Corbis: Tim Pannell. 129 Masterfile: Kevin Dodge. 142 Getty Images: Stone/Claudia Kunin. 143 Corbis: Larry Williams. 144 Corbis: photocuisine/Roulier/Turiot. 152 Getty Images: Iconica/Tom Grill. 153 Corbis: Richard Cummins (l). 162 Corbis: Fabio Cardoso. 166 Corbis: Ariel Skelley. 170 Getty Images: Iconica/Zia Soleil. 176 SuperStock: Stuart Pearce. 180 Corbis: George Shelley

All other images © Dorling Kindersley
For further information see: www.dkimages.com